MARGIN OVER MISSION

MARGIN OVER MISSION

When Private Equity Owns Your Hospital

JAMES KELLY, RN

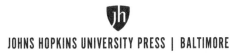

JOHNS HOPKINS UNIVERSITY PRESS | BALTIMORE

© 2025 Johns Hopkins University Press
All rights reserved. Published 2025
Printed in the United States of America on acid-free paper
9   8   7   6   5   4   3   2   1

Johns Hopkins University Press
2715 North Charles Street
Baltimore, Maryland 21218
www.press.jhu.edu

Library of Congress Cataloging-in-Publication Data

Names: Kelly, James, 1948– author.
Title: Margin over mission : when private equity owns your hospital /
    James Kelly, RN.
Description: Baltimore : Johns Hopkins University Press, 2025. |
    Includes bibliographical references and index.
Identifiers: LCCN 2024033465 | ISBN 9781421451459 (hardcover ; alk. paper) |
    ISBN 9781421451466 (ebook)
Subjects: MESH: Lovelace Women's Hospital. | Hospitals, Proprietary—
    economics | Women's Health Services—economics | Quality of Health Care—
    trends | Hospital Mortality—trends | Failure to Rescue, Health Care—trends |
    Private Sector—economics | New Mexico | Personal Narrative
Classification: LCC RA971 | NLM WX 28 AN5 | DDC 362.11068—
    dc23/eng/20240814
LC record available at https://lccn.loc.gov/2024033465

A catalog record for this book is available from the British Library.

Special discounts are available for bulk purchases of this book. For more information,
please contact Special Sales at specialsales@jh.edu.

To Loren, for all the miles and all the years

CONTENTS

MARGIN OVER MISSION

Prologue

"Hi, my name is Jim Kelly. I'll be your nurse today." I've said that thousands of times over 22 years of being an ICU nurse. I've said it to Hispanics, Anglos, Navajo; to Pueblo Indians, Hopi, and Apache; to the young and the old; to the calm, the delirious, the terrified, and the angry. I've said it in New Mexico, California, Oregon, and Arizona. The last time I'll say it will be in the ICU at Lovelace Women's Hospital across from the Rock & Brews on Montgomery Boulevard in the city where it all began: Albuquerque, New Mexico.

A career is a life of learning, a mastery of craft. I remember my first year in nursing. Everything was new; everything was the first time. I was working nights in the ICU at St. Joseph's Hospital in Albuquerque. I would drive home up I-25 to Santa Fe. Before I went to bed, I would look up why phenylephrine causes reflex bradycardia or why we use vasopressin in septic shock. On days off, I read the book all the residents had: *The ICU Book*, by Paul Marino. At work, at the beginning of every shift, I thought about my patient's diagnosis, about what could happen and what I would do if it happened. Over the years, I learned what to do. I felt I had mastered my craft.

A hospital is a separate world. The ICU is a separate world within it. The suffering. The fear of loss. The fight to live. The deaths. In his book *Moderated Love: A Theology of Professional Care*, Alastair Campbell writes that we should think of nursing as companionship. Companionship is closeness but it is less than friendship. It's a journey. The good companion helps with the journey, travels along until the journey ends and the companions part ways.[1] I think of all the patients and families I have been companion to over the years. Some journeys were longer than others. Some ended in sadness. But I came to feel that every day, for the 12 hours I was in the ICU, I was at the heart of things.

Yet my career didn't end with a feeling of fulfillment, of gratitude for the many years in nursing. It ended in discord, and I felt alienated from the hospital, suffering a loss of faith in leadership. My last year in nursing felt like a world different from the one I had been working in for 22 years. I wondered: Had it been there all along and I didn't realize it, or was it something new? It began with a patient dying who shouldn't have. Then another. And another. Preventable deaths. They seemed random. Like stars coming out in the evening sky. Then I realized they weren't random. They were connected. There was a pattern. A constellation. Orion. Andromeda.

It felt like we had betrayed our mission as a community hospital, broken our covenant with the people of Albuquerque. I wondered why decisions were being made—clinical, administrative—that led to the deaths of patients. I wondered about Lovelace. Where did the name come from? When I worked in the downtown hospital in 1998, it was St. Joseph's. In 2005 it was Albuquerque Regional Medical Center. A year later it was Lovelace Medical Center. Before it was Lovelace Women's Hospital, it was Northeast Heights. Was there something in names, something in the past to explain things? I knew we were owned by a company called Ardent Health Services. That it was based in Nashville. I found a book: *The Lovelace Medical Center: Pioneer in American Health Care*.[2] It was written by Jake Spidle, a professor in the history department at the University of New Mexico. It was a thread that slowly unraveled the mystery, explained what happened and why.

I began to write. You write to understand. Annie Dillard says, "When you write, you lay out a line of words. The line of words is a miner's pick, a woodcarver's gouge, a surgeon's probe. You wield it and it digs a path you follow. Soon you find yourself deep in new territory."[3] Before I wrote this book, I didn't know about leveraged buyouts, OpCo/PropCo deals, dividend recapitalization, tax arbitrage. I didn't know who Randy Lovelace was. I found them on the path.

The story of the Lovelace Health System in New Mexico is the story of an institution that began with one man and a vision of service, of a mission-driven hospital that became a transcendent medical presence in the Southwest. It is also a story of fallen glory, of how that vision died in the hands of Wall Street.

In "'Murder Most Foul' and the Haunting of America," Timothy Hampton's review of Bob Dylan's song about the assassination of John F. Kennedy, the author talks about the struggle in American literature to grasp and comprehend larger political and economic forces and the spiritual and moral changes in daily life wrought by them. Artists, Hampton writes, are sometimes able to grasp these forces through "small flakes of experience which gestured—allegorically, as it were—to the larger catastrophes of our national life. The small towns of Faulkner, the paranoid communities of Pynchon, the tangled but discrete 'cases' of Raymond Chandler, all reflect beyond themselves onto the guilt, corruption, and greed that power our national political 'progress' and economic 'growth.'"[4]

This book is about my last year in nursing, a small flake of experience.

1

The Covenant

Being a nurse in a hospital also means being a nurse in a town or a city. They're connected. Hospitals and cities grow up together. When the population increases, the hospital adds a wing. When the city expands, the hospital follows it with clinics. A hospital is woven into the lives of the people of the city. It's where you were born, where you had children, where family members were ill, where some of them died. Charles Rosenberg describes America's hospital system as the care of strangers.[1] Being a nurse in a hospital in a city involves caring for strangers with whom you share a place, a history, traditions, memories. Strangers you are loyal to and responsible for. Strangers you treat like family.

In his book of the same title, V. B. Price, a columnist for the *Albuquerque Tribune*, calls Albuquerque the "city at the end of the world" because of its geographic isolation—the seventeenth-century conquistador Diego de Vargas called it "remote beyond compare"—and because, as the capital of America's nuclear war machine, it would be one of the first targets in a nuclear war.[2] In 1947, the Atomic Energy Commission took over Sandia Base and established the Armed Forces Special Weapons Project for the maintenance, storage, security, and handling of nuclear weapons. The Kirtland Underground Munitions Maintenance and Storage Complex, completed in 1994, is the largest storage facility for nuclear weapons in the world. Tunnels in the foothills of the Manzano Mountains contain 2,450 nuclear warheads.

Price describes Albuquerque as a full-fledged, mainstream American city in the middle of a natural wilderness, the high desert plateau of central New Mexico bordered to the east by the Sandia and Manzano Mountains and to the west by the fourth-longest river in North America, the Rio Grande, and its bosque woodlands.

It's a city grappling with modern problems. In 2021, for the third year in a row, New Mexico posted the third-highest poverty rate in the country at 18.4%. New Mexico also had the third-highest poverty rate in the country for residents younger than 18 years of age at 23.9%.[3] Nearly a sixth (16.2%) of the population of Albuquerque lives below the poverty line.[4] Albuquerque is one of the most violent cities in the country. In 2021, there were a record-breaking 117 homicides.[5] The violent crime is largely drug fueled. For years New Mexico has had the highest or second-highest rate of overdose deaths in the country. In 2018, the FBI declared the Albuquerque Metropolitan Area the robbery capital of the United States. A report by the US Department of Housing and Urban Development found that from 2018 to 2019, New Mexico had a 27% increase in homelessness, the largest in the nation. The 57.6% increase in chronic homelessness was also the largest in the nation. Albuquerque's homeless population rose by 15%. It is estimated that 3,000 children enrolled in Albuquerque public schools are considered homeless at any given time over the course of a school year.[6]

In a 2018 white paper on the opioid crisis, the National Safety Council found that New Mexico was one of only three states to adopt all of its recommended actions, including mandating continuing education for doctors prescribing opioids; requiring drug overdose data to be reported; and making naloxone, the opioid overdose reversal drug, widely available. It was the first state with statewide syringe services, the first state to have an overdose prevention program, the first to pass a Good Samaritan law. On April 6, 2021, Albuquerque mayor Tim Keller announced that the city had bought a 572,000-square-foot complex for $15 million and would transform it into a gateway center for the homeless that would provide primary care, behavioral health services, and shelter.[7] The City of Albuquerque developed one of the largest community land trust projects in the United States. Arbolera de Vida (Orchard of Life) is 27 acres of reclaimed industrial property transformed into a community-designed, mixed-use, urban infill project for low- to moderate-income New Mexican families that offers affordable homes, senior housing, civic spaces, and employment opportunities.

The city has a unique spiritual and cultural heritage. The historical Hispanic culture of Albuquerque is surrounded by nineteen pueblo villages that continue Indigenous spiritual traditions that began 2,000 years ago. It's a city of neighborhoods, havens that offer refuge from the vastness of the desert, from "old Hispanic strongholds like Atrisco, Pajarito, and Barelas in the South Valley; Duranes, Santa Barbara Martíneztown, San José in the mid Valley; [and] John Marshall, an Afro-American enclave on South Broadway near downtown" to "historic areas such as the Victorian Huning-Highland neighborhood" and "the turn-of-the-century Midwestern Downtown Neighborhood."[8]

It is culturally diverse. Anglos, Native New Mexican Hispanics, Mexican Americans, Hispanics of pure Spanish descent, and mestizos of Spanish and Indigenous background. Navajo. Apache. Pueblo Indians with their three distinct languages: Keres, Zuni, and Tanoan. The Gathering of Nations is the largest pow-wow in North America. It's held annually on the fourth weekend in April at Expo NM in Albuquerque. It draws over 700 tribes from the United States and Canada.

Sixty miles north of Albuquerque, the exotic city of Santa Fe is the political capital of the state. In 1880, the Atchison, Topeka and Santa Fe Railway bypassed Santa Fe and arrived in Albuquerque, setting the two cities on paths to different destinies. Santa Fe embraced the romantic historical image of New Mexico. It became an art colony and a cultural mecca. It attracted tourists and an affluent real estate clientele. National media described Santa Fe as the "Tahiti in the desert."[9]

Albuquerque became a metropolis of over half a million people. It's a university town, the home of a medical school, and the business capital of the state. Within a three-mile radius of downtown Albuquerque are five hospitals: the University of New Mexico Hospital (UNM) on Lomas, Presbyterian on Cedar, Lovelace Medical Center (LMC) on Martin Luther King Jr. Boulevard, Heart Hospital on Elm, and Lovelace Women's Hospital.

Women's Hospital is at 4701 Montgomery Boulevard NE. Albuquerque is divided into four unequal quadrants: the dividing lines are the east–west Central Avenue and the north–south railroad tracks. Central Avenue was originally part of Route 66. In *The Grapes of Wrath*, John Steinbeck called it the "Mother Road." Addresses north of Central and east of the railroad tracks are designated "NE." Across from the hospital on Montgomery, the Rock & Brews sign says the restaurant sells scratch-prepared American comfort food and craft beer. Behind it is a big Smith's grocery. To the west of the hospital, you can see the calderas of the West Mesa; to the east, the Sandia Mountains.

Women's ICU is only eight beds. They're on the left when you walk in, numbered backward from 232 to 225. We have three categories of patients in descending acuity: ICU status, Intermediate Care (IMC), and Medical-Surgical (Med-Surg). Unlike most ICUs, we admit IMC patients. The patient–nurse ratio for ICU status is two to one; for IMC, three to one; and for Med-Surg, four to one. ICU vital signs are taken every hour; IMC every four. Some days, we have no ICU patients. We can go months without a patient on a ventilator. Even longer without a code. But we have a unique place in the landscape of health care in the state. "Lovelace Women's Hospital is New Mexico's first and only hospital dedicated to women's health and features a 53-bed Level III Neonatal Intensive Care Unit, . . . 16 labor and delivery rooms, [a] 41-bed Mother-Baby unit, [and] a Maternal-Fetal Medicine program for high-risk pregnancies."[10] There's the GRACE program—Giving Respect and Compassion to Expecting Moms—for pregnant women and their families living with substance use or addiction, including opioids and heroin, because many mothers are addicted and give birth to babies that are addicted.

We're one of the smaller hospitals in Albuquerque. We're a destination but we're also a tributary. If you're dying, we can save your life. But if there's something we can't do—cardiac catheterization, interventional radiology, neurosurgery—we'll send you somewhere that can, to UNM, Heart, LMC. It's our covenant with the people of Albuquerque.

Lovelace Women's Hospital isn't a Level 1 trauma center like UNM. It's not Presbyterian, with hospitals all over the state. But it's one thing they're not: it's owned by a private equity firm.

2

Lovelace, 1922–1991

The New Mexican historian Erna Fergusson wrote that, at the turn of the century, Albuquerque had only two industries, the Santa Fe railroad and tuberculosis.[1] The White Plague claimed 150,000 lives in the United States every year. In the middle of the nineteenth century, a new treatment emerged: "altitude therapy." At first a trickle, then a stream, of the afflicted flowed into the Rocky Mountain West and New Mexico chasing the cure of sunshine and pristine air. Scientists theorized a level in the atmosphere free of germs and suffused with heat, light, and electricity that resisted tuberculosis. It was thought to be approximately 5,000 feet above sea level. It was called the Line of Immunity.[2] New Mexico was called the "Well Country."[3]

The migration not only populated the state with tuberculars from the East Coast and Midwest, it shaped the future of medicine in New Mexico. It laid the foundation for the development of hospitals in the state. Between 1865 and 1937, there were 31 sanatoria in New Mexico. Over the years, the migration slowed and the sanatoria were transformed into hospitals: Albuquerque's Presbyterian Medical Center, St. Vincent's in Santa Fe, St. Mary's in

Roswell. It was the main reason for the influx of hundreds of physicians. From 1885 to 1910, the number of physicians quadrupled. Most of them had tuberculosis and were seeking their own cure in the high desert. They were young doctors who would never have thought of practicing in the frontier wilderness of New Mexico. One of them was a 23-year-old from Belle, Missouri, who arrived in Sunnyside, New Mexico, in April 1906. His name was William Randolph Lovelace.

Before leaving Missouri, Dr. Lovelace had arranged with authorities of the Santa Fe railroad and the Lantry Sharp Construction Company, which was laying railroad tracks across eastern New Mexico to Kansas, to work as the railroad and company surgeon at their Sunnyside railroad camp. A 1908 photograph shows the profile of the young doctor in his cabin-sized office, seated next to a cylindrical wood stove. His back is to a desk. He is facing a shelved wall of medications. Country doctors were their own pharmacists.

After equipping his office, Dr. Lovelace had nothing in the bank and $8 in cash. He also had an Iver Johnson revolver he had purchased for $2.50 before he left St. Louis. Years later, he would say it was a "comforting possession" as he traveled day and night on long buggy rides through the Pecos Valley wilderness. Not long after he arrived, he had a severe setback, a siege of pulmonary hemorrhaging. His mother, Edna, came to nurse him back to health. Within two years, the whole family from Missouri had moved to Sunnyside: his father, John L. Lovelace; two younger sisters, Maybelle and Lora; his older brother, Edgar, and Edgar's wife, Jewell, and their six-month-old son, William Randolph Lovelace II.

He served not only the railroad but the town and a large part of the surrounding Pecos Valley countryside. He traveled the arid landscape of the high plains delivering a baby for a sheepherder's wife, caring for a child with scarlet fever, setting the leg of a ranch hand. He was known for his devotion to his patients, his solicitude for their well-being. Ever willing to help, kind to the rich and poor, he was revered. The Spanish-speaking people would say, "Despues de Dios, el Doctor."[4] In 1913 he moved to Albuquerque, looking, as he would write at the age of 86, for a "place to serve."[5]

In 1918, Edgar Lassetter, who had contracted tuberculosis while in military service in the Philippines during the Spanish-American War and received treatment at the army sanitarium in Fort Bayard, moved to Albuquerque from Georgia. He met Dr. Lovelace through the doctor's younger sister Lora, whom he would marry in 1919. That year, they merged their practices, and in 1922 they started a formal partnership. Although the designation was first used in 1929, that year is considered the birth of the Lovelace Clinic. They shared a strong commitment to patient care. Dr. Lassetter, Jake Spidle writes, "possessed the special compassion and dedication associated with the best among the old-time country doctors and general practitioners. He was devoted to his patients and both Drs. Lovelace and Lassetter became legendary for their attentiveness to their patients."[6] House calls were a central part of their practice. At night, when the clinic switchboard was closed, the clinic's telephone number rang in Dr. Lovelace's home. One young doctor whom Dr. Lovelace had called to attend to Mrs. Ortega, who had a bellyache, accidentally fell asleep and was awakened by the taxicab sent to his house by Dr. Lovelace.[7]

The Mayo Clinic in Rochester, Minnesota, was considered the lodestar of American medicine. At a time when American physicians were committed to the tradition of individual practice, Mayo was pioneering the concept of multispecialty group practice with board-certified specialists in surgery; obstetrics and gynecology; radiology; pediatrics; internal medicine; and ear, nose, and throat. Dr. Lovelace made annual trips to the clinic. He became a lifelong friend of the Mayo brothers, Drs. Will and Charlie. It became his dream to establish a Mayo-type institution in the Southwest.

In the late 1920s, Drs. Lovelace and Lassetter made the decision to expand their partnership into a group practice. It grew slowly from the two founders in 1929, to five physicians in 1932, and ten in 1939. The specialties were pediatrics; radiology; ear, nose, and throat; internal medicine; and urology. By 1941, the clinic numbered 14 physicians, making it the largest concentration of medical manpower in the Southwest and a regional referral center. The Lovelace Clinic joined Seattle's Mason Clinic, founded in 1920; the Cleveland Clinic (1921); and the Lahey Clinic in Boston (1923) as trailblazers in the group-practice movement in American medicine.

In 1947, Dr. Lovelace's nephew, William Randolph "Randy" Lovelace II, joined the clinic and would, by force of his vision, energy, and talent, transform it and elevate it to national prominence. He began his career in a surgery fellowship at the Mayo Clinic in Rochester in 1936. In 1940, he was appointed first assistant to Charles Mayo and in 1941 was designated a Mayo surgical chief. At Mayo, he came under the influence of Walter M. Boothby, one of the pioneers of aviation medicine. Drs. Boothby and Randy Lovelace, together with Arthur H. Bulbulian, invented the BLB mask, named for its inventors, an oxygen mask for high-altitude flight to combat the risk of hypoxia. Randy Lovelace personally tested it in flights as high as 15,000 feet. The BLB mask became standard equipment in military and commercial aircraft.

During World War II Lovelace was assigned to a research position at the Aero Medical Laboratory at Wright Field, Ohio, and was chief of the laboratory's Oxygen Branch, where he focused on the dangers of bailout at high altitudes. He and his team designed a small bailout cylinder that contained a 12-minute supply of oxygen. It needed to be tested. On June 24, 1943, Lovelace parachuted from a B-17 at 40,200 feet above the wheat fields of central Washington State. The air temperature was 50 degrees below zero. The initial blast of air and the jolt of the parachute opening—

four times greater at 40,000 feet than at sea level—tore the glove off his left hand and knocked him unconscious. He regained consciousness 15 minutes later at 8,000 feet. He landed in a field of wheat stubble. He had severe frostbite on the gloveless hand and was nauseated from swinging to and fro while unconscious, but the oxygen bottle had worked. There were pictures and articles about the event in *Life* and *Look* magazines. It was the first and only parachute jump of his life.

After his military duty, Lovelace returned to the Mayo Clinic. In the summer of 1946, Rochester was struck by a polio epidemic. On July 7, the Lovelaces' five-and-a-half-year-old son, William Randolph Lovelace III, died. Three weeks later, their other son, four-year-old Chuckie Lovelace died. Later that year, the Lovelaces left Rochester and moved to Albuquerque, and Randy Lovelace became a full partner with his two uncles, inaugurating a golden age of the Lovelace Clinic.

In 1947, opportunities for medical education were virtually nonexistent in the American Southwest. From Dallas–Fort Worth to Los Angeles and from Denver to the Mexican border, there was not one medical school; no hospitals with approved internship or residency programs; very few nursing schools; not a single program for the training of medical personnel such as X-ray or lab technicians, physical therapists, or dietitians. Imbued with his experience at Mayo, Randy Lovelace envisioned a modern medical foundation in the Southwest based on the triad of medical care, education, and research.

On September 24, 1947, after months of legal work and close liaison with Mayo, the Lovelace Foundation for Medical Education and Research was formally incorporated. It consisted of five physicians and nine laymen. Its purposes were defined as educational, scientific, benevolent, and charitable.

Not only had the clinic outgrown its offices on two floors of the First National Bank building in downtown Albuquerque, but additional space was needed for the new physicians, laboratories, and research personnel of the Lovelace Foundation. In October 1950, on land donated by William Lovelace, the Lovelace Clinic Building on Gibson Boulevard in southeast Albuquerque had its grand opening. Charles Mayo was the chief speaker. The 50,000-square-foot structure, four stories high, pueblo style, was designed by esteemed Southwest architect John Gaw Meem. For the next 35 years, the Clinic Building, or Building 1—the names by which it was known—remained the heart of the Lovelace Clinic. Over the next decade it would expand by over 80,000 square feet, adding a 7,500-square-foot Radiation Therapy Center in 1953 and a 5,000-square-foot OB-GYN building in 1961. When Randy Lovelace joined the clinic in 1946, it comprised a dozen physicians with specialties in internal medicine, general surgery, pediatrics, radiology, and obstetrics and gynecology. Three years later, the staff had grown to nearly 30 physicians in 16 areas. In the following decade, it doubled to more than 60. National media praised the progressive medical center: "Medicine at Its Best" (*Los Angeles Daily News*, May 6, 1952); "Selfless Docs" (*New York World Telegram*, April 30, 1952).[8]

Although it focused on serving a general, local practice, it was the largest single concentration of medical manpower and expertise for hundreds of miles, it was a specialty referral center for a broad portion of the Rocky Mountain region, and it exercised a powerful influence over the practice and development of medicine throughout the Southwest.

In April 1952, the 104-bed Bataan Memorial Methodist Hospital—named for the New Mexico soldiers of the 200th Army Coast Artillery who fought in the World War II battle and endured the death march—opened on land adjacent to the one-year-old Lovelace Clinic. Although it wasn't purchased by the Lovelace Medical Foundation until October 1969, from its very inception it was an integral part of Lovelace. It was referred to as "the clinic's hospital." Over a decade later, it had expanded to 245 beds and was admitting 8,500 patients a year. It had a record of innovation. Its history includes a long list of firsts. In 1957, it opened the state's first intensive-care unit. In 1959, it performed the first open-heart surgery in New Mexico and, in the same year, the first kidney dialysis. It was the first American hospital with a heart-lung resuscitator and the nation's first cystic fibrosis research and treatment center. In 1971, it became the world's first hospital to perform a lung lavage procedure to flush radioactive particles from a patient's lungs.[9]

The Lovelace Foundation's research efforts began slowly in late 1947–1948. The foundation's annual research report for 1950–1951 showed a focus on aviation medicine. In 1952, Randy Lovelace arranged a groundbreaking symposium to plan and coordinate research on manned flight to the top of the atmosphere. It attracted national and international scientists—astrophysicists, biologists, aviation medicine specialists—and established the Lovelace Foundation as a major research center for aviation medicine. The proceedings of the symposium were published as *Physics and Medicine of the Upper Atmosphere* and became a classic work in that field.

A 1951 contract with the Atomic Energy Commission (AEC) provided financial impetus to the foundation's research program. The blast and shock biology program, which would last 35 years, was authorized by the AEC's Division of Biology and Medicine in the aftermath of the Hiroshima and Nagasaki atomic bombs. Unlike other research centers in the country, which studied the thermal and radiation effects of nuclear explosions, the Lovelace program focused on the biological consequences of high-yield explosions and the damage produced by energized debris. The $4 million contract allowed the foundation to expand staff and purchase sophisticated equipment. It produced over 90 scientific studies in the first 15 years. The program was a collaborative effort at the foundation, reflecting its ethos of cooperation. The clinic departments involved were the Departments of Comparative Environmental Biology, Engineering, Pathology, and Physics. Supporting departments were the Departments of Biomathematics and Computer Systems, Medical Illustration, and Veterinary Medicine and the library.

In the 1950s, the AEC was concerned with the potential health effects of radiation and the toxicity that might be encountered in the development, manufacture, testing, and possible use of nuclear weapons, as well as in the growing nuclear power industry. In 1961, the AEC's Division of Biology and Medicine contracted with the Lovelace Clinic to develop a program to evaluate the hazards of the release of radioactive fission products into the environment and the effect of radionuclides that might be inhaled and deposited in the body. New departments of aerosol physics and radiobiology were established, and the Departments of Biochemistry, Microbiology, and Pathology were expanded to support the research. The program, called the Fission Product Inhalation Program, grew quickly to 24 full-time scientific and engineering professionals, a corps of technical and support personnel, and a budget of $1.7 million. The first scholarly papers appeared in 1962.

Clinical research at the foundation developed more slowly. The Lovelace Clinic staff were engaged in clinical studies, but they were also practicing physicians. Lovelace physicians dedicated a portion of their time without compensation to clinical projects. Research did occur in the areas of cancer therapy, infant resuscitation equipment and techniques, and therapeutic agents for the treatment of arthritis. The first major clinical research project, supported by a 1962 National Institutes of Health grant, was the cardiovascular research program, which focused on the development of equipment and new techniques for cardiac surgery and cardiopulmonary resuscitation, including the use of deep hypothermia. The project produced over 20 scientific papers, two prize-winning educational and training videos, and several training sessions on heart-lung resuscitation that were conducted at the local, state, and national levels.

The third component of Randy Lovelace's vision—education—took more time to develop. The 1958–1959 annual report broached the idea of the foundation forming its own medical school. It was dissuaded from it by the burgeoning momentum for a state-supported school at the University of New Mexico, which opened in 1964. By 1965, the educational mission of the foundation was in full bloom. There were five approved residency programs—internal medicine, surgery, radiology, pathology, and aerospace medicine—open to 25 residents; an externship program for medical students, which brought medical students to the Lovelace-Bataan facilities from such schools as the University of Oklahoma School of Medicine, Philadelphia's Jefferson Medical College, and the Louisiana State University School of Medicine; a postgraduate fellowship program; and a school for X-ray technology approved by the American Medical Association's Council on Medical Education. The Lovelace Clinic also continued to provide a site for the rotation of nursing students from local schools.

As Randy Lovelace was ascendant, Uncle Doc, as William Lovelace became known, took a lesser role but continued to work into his 80s. He continued to emphasize to Randy the importance of the clinic in the larger Lovelace scheme, stressing "at every opportunity the old-time ethic of taking care of the patient first and foremost" and "the indispensability of personalized patient care of the highest quality possible."[10]

In 1958, the most prestigious event in the Lovelace Foundation's history occurred and elevated it to national prominence in the field of aviation and aerospace medicine. Since the late 1940s, the Lovelace Foundation and Clinic had been involved in the clinical examination of airline- and aviation-industry test pilots and in aviation medicine research. In 1958, a newly created federal agency, NASA, announced its first major undertaking. Project Mercury would launch the first national manned space capsule into orbit around the earth. The Lovelace Foundation was asked to assume responsibility for the testing and medical selection of the first group of American astronauts who would fly in Project Mercury. There were 32 astronaut aspirants. In February 1959, the Lovelace Foundation began testing the first of six groups. The testing period lasted seven and a half days and three evenings. Seven astronauts were selected. They would be known as the Mercury 7.

On December 12, 1965, Randy and Mary Lovelace, with their pilot Milton Brown, left Aspen, Colorado, in a Beechcraft Travelair for the two-hour flight to Albuquerque. They had been in Aspen looking at a condominium they were building and visiting Alvin Eurich, a member of the Lovelace Foundation's board of trustees. A half hour into the flight, the plane crashed in a mountain canyon. All three aboard were killed. It took searchers three days, moving through deep snow, to reach the crash site. It was the same day of the rendezvous in deep space of Gemini 6 and Gemini 7, an irony noted by President Lyndon Johnson, who, in an official statement, acknowledged Randy Lovelace's contributions to and enduring legacy in space medicine. All seven Mercury astronauts returned for the funeral.[11] In 1970, NASA announced that a crater on the moon had been named in honor of William Randolph Lovelace II. William Randolph Lovelace died three years later in 1968 at age 85.

Despite the loss of both its founder and its visionary force, over the next two decades the Lovelace Clinic remained faithful to its founding principles of health care, medical research, and medical education and true to its pioneering spirit.

In the 1970s, the city grew away from the clinic on Southeast Gibson toward the West Mesa and the Northeast Heights. Concerned that patients might not be willing to travel the increased distance, the clinic decided to go to them. It expanded beyond Gibson with a string of satellite clinics. The first satellite clinic opened in Rio Rancho in May 1975. Two years later, a second satellite clinic opened on Juan Tabo in the Northeast Heights. The Rio Rancho clinic saw fewer than 6,000 patients in its inaugural year; in 1985, it saw 200,000. By 1987 there were seven satellite clinics throughout the city. A large percentage of patients who visited the satellites were seeking care for problems outside the internist's expertise. This led Lovelace to embrace the new and modern specialty called family practice. By 1986, 34 of the 151 staff physicians were family-medicine practitioners.

Lovelace established the first health maintenance organization (HMO) in the Southwest. The Lovelace Health Plan, as it was named, grew from 3,600 members in 1980 to 69,800 in 1986. Lovelace, Spidle writes, "had established itself as both a regional and national leader in the reshaping of the structure of the American health-care delivery system near the end of the twentieth century."[12]

The death of Randy Lovelace led to a fading of the emphasis on aviation medicine. Under the influence of the environmental movement in the 1970s, the inhalation toxicology program moved beyond the focus on radionuclides to a broad array of chemical toxicants inhaled by people in their everyday life, from aerosolized consumer products to diesel exhaust emissions. The program worked with the National Institutes of Health, the US Food and Drug Administration, and the Consumer Product Safety Commission. In 1973, the name of the Fission Product Inhalation Program was changed to the Inhalation Toxicology Research Institute. By 1980, the institute had a staff of 50 doctoral-level specialists and 190 support personnel and a budget of $11.5 million. In the mid-1980s, it produced 80–100 scholarly papers a year. Graduate students at both the master's and doctoral degree levels conducted thesis and dissertation research at the institute, and 10–12 pursued postdoctoral studies every year.

Other research was being conducted in the Clinical Research Division. Studies involved noninvasive blood flow investigations using Doppler echocardiography; research on connective tissue disease, especially arthritis; identification of markers for DNA damage and repair; and immunodiagnostics. In 1984, the division was awarded a three-year, $36 million contract to study the effects of Agent Orange exposure on Vietnam veterans.

In 1976, David J. Ottensmeyer, a neurosurgeon, became president and chief executive officer of the Lovelace Medical Center. He vastly increased the satellite clinic program, recruited a new generation of young physicians, and oversaw the blossoming of the Lovelace HMO, but he also did something not done in the six-decade history of Lovelace: he surrendered the independence and autonomy of the institution.

In the mid-1980s, Lovelace experienced a financial challenge in the aging and decay of Bataan Hospital. The hospital had been built to standards of the 1940s, and attempts at renovation and repair that had to adhere to building, fire, and safety codes of the 1980s were proving to be prohibitively expensive. The $45 million cost of a new hospital far exceeded the assets of the foundation and led Lovelace to contemplate abandoning its historical "stand alone" policy and look for a financial partner. After negotiations with Presbyterian Hospital failed to develop, Lovelace began discussion with several regional and national health-care companies on a possible partnership.

The concern of the Lovelace community was preserving the uniqueness of the institution and the integrity of the research and education programs. Ottensmeyer sought to address this concern in a report to the Lovelace Foundation Board of Trustees in March 1984 that delineated the objectives that would guide Lovelace's bargaining with outside companies. The report assured

that the Lovelace Medical Foundation would have sufficient resources and revenue to carry on activities central to its missions
and goals, medical education and research would be integrated
with health-care delivery in any new organization, the foundation
would have 50% representation on the board of directors, and the
jobs of the foundation's medical staff and employees would be
secure.

In June 1984, the Lovelace Board of Trustees approved a joint
venture partnership with the for-profit health-industry giant Hospital Corporation of America (HCA) that would create a new entity called the Lovelace Medical Center, Inc. The agreement gave
HCA 80% equity and the Lovelace Medical Foundation 20%. The
foundation secured the right to name 50% of the board of directors and approve the CEO. HCA would go on to build a new
$43 million 243-bed hospital on Gibson. Lovelace would have its
debt liquidated.[13]

In Lovelace's 1984 annual report, Dr. Ottensmeyer argued that
it was a bold move but consistent with "'the tradition of enterprise
and innovation that have characterized Lovelace since the days
of Randy Lovelace and Uncle Doc.' Building on that foundation,
Lovelace stood poised to meet the challenges at the end of the
twentieth century."[14]

In truth, the apprehensions of the Lovelace community were
prescient. In October 1986, Lovelace fell into the hands of another corporate giant of the health-care world, the Equitable
Life Assurance Society of the United States. HCA and Equitable entered into a joint venture to form a new company called
Equicor, which would offer managed health care and other
employee benefit programs on a national scale. The new company was formed by combining HCA's Health Plan Division, of
which the Lovelace Health Plan was a part, and the Equitable
Group and Health Insurance Company Division of the insurance company.

Ottensmeyer left Albuquerque for Nashville to become senior vice president of HCA. In 1990, Connecticut-based insurance behemoth Cigna bought HCA's 80% share of the company and then bought the remaining 20% in 1991. At the turn of the century, Lovelace would fall deeper into the corporate world.

3

Private Equity

Private equity firms are Wall Street investment firms that pool large volumes of capital from investors such as pension funds, mutual funds, and sovereign wealth funds (e.g., Norway Government Pension Fund), and wealthy individuals to buy companies. "Private" means they're not traded on the US stock market. If private equity acquires control of a public company, it "takes it private," delisting it from the public stock exchange.

Private equity has its origins in the leveraged buyout (LBO) movement of the 1980s, known as the Decade of Greed. It was commonly associated with "hostile takeovers" and "corporate raiders." Acquisitions were unwelcome, unsolicited, and destabilizing. After his hostile takeover of TWA in 1985, Carl Icahn sold TWA's assets to repay the debt he used to purchase the company. Almost half of US public corporations experienced a takeover attempt in that decade. The LBO movement ended in 1990 with a record number of companies acquired in LBOs filing for bankruptcy. Drexel Burnham Lambert, the investment bank most responsible for the boom in LBOs, pleaded guilty to six felonies. Junk bond inventor Michael Milken was sentenced to 10 years in prison, fined $600 million, and permanently barred from the securities industry by the Securities and Exchange Commission. The excesses of the period were chronicled in the book and later the HBO movie *Barbarians at the Gate*, which examine the $25 billion takeover of RJR Nabisco by the American global investment firm Kohlberg Kravis Roberts (KKR). Burdened by debt, the company was broken up and 2,000 workers lost their jobs. The LBO model of the 1980s was discredited and viewed as dead.

LBOs reemerged in the late 1990s with a new degree of legitimacy and respectability. Over the past two decades the private equity industry has grown from $700 billion in global assets to $5.8 trillion. Today, private equity owns or operates twice as many companies as are publicly traded on the US stock market. The private equity industry owns hospitals, restaurants, retailers, for-profit colleges, payday lenders, nursing homes, trailer parks, hospices, prisons, casinos, golf courses, and newspapers.

In an LBO, a company is purchased with a large amount of borrowed money, referred to as debt. The acquired company is called the portfolio company. The outside investors are called the limited partners. The limited partners are passive investors who have no decision-making authority. The managers of the private equity firm are called the general partners. Traditionally, firms use a combination of debt and equity to finance a transaction. The capital structure of a publicly traded company is typically 30% debt and 70% equity. Private equity is the opposite: 70% debt and 30% equity. The limited partners provide 20%–30% equity; the general partners 1%–2%. The remaining 70% is borrowed money, usually from a bank loan. In 2000, Mitt Romney's Bain Capital performed an LBO of KB Toys. Bain put down $18 million in equity for the $304 million buyout and leveraged the rest: 6% equity and 94% debt.[1]

The personal funds invested by the general partners are a small fraction of the purchase price of the companies the fund acquires.

They can use as little as 0.05% of their own funds on massive, multimillion-dollar transactions. Debt magnifies the return to the private equity fund. When the company is sold to another firm or taken public, the lion's share of the gains is captured by the private equity general partners. General partners typically receive 20% of profits above a threshold rate of 8% given to the limited partners. "Leveraging amplifies possible returns, just like a lever can be used to amplify one's strength when moving a heavy weight."[2] The general partners can put in a comparatively small amount of cash but accrue considerable profit when they sell. They "leverage" their small investment into outsize returns. The general partners have little at stake if debt drives the acquired company into bankruptcy but much to gain from a successful exit from the investment. Debt is the lifeblood of private equity. Little to lose, much to gain.

The acquired company—not the private equity firm—is responsible for repaying the debt and the interest on it. High debt levels put pressure on the portfolio company's managers to cut costs in order to boost profits and thus meet debt obligations. Saddled by debt, companies can lose the capacity to invest, innovate, increase compensation for workers, or respond to a changing economic environment such as e-commerce.

Workers invariably pay the price for private equity takeovers. A 2019 study by researchers at Harvard Business School and the University of Chicago that analyzed almost 10,000 LBOs between 1980 and 2013 found significant job loss following private equity takeovers. The report found average job losses of 4.4% in the two years after a company was bought by private equity. Employment fell by 13% when a private equity firm took over a publicly traded company. In addition, average earnings per worker fell by 1.7% after a buyout.[3] Profits are taken from workers not only through layoffs—which intensify work for those who remain—but also in myriad other ways: lowering wages, eliminating raises, reducing benefits like health care and retirement, eliminating severance payments, replacing employee pensions with a 401(k) plan that has no employer match or contribution, and discontinuing reimbursement programs covering employee education.

"Leverage" refers not only to the use of debt and but also to the amount of debt a firm has taken on. A company that is "highly leveraged" has more debt than equity. When it is "overleveraged," it is carrying too much debt relative to its earnings. An overleveraged company has difficulty paying the interest and principal on the debt and is often unable to pay its operating expenses. This can lead to a downward financial spiral. The company has to borrow more capital to stay in operation, and the problem gets worse. This spiral usually ends when a company restructures its debt or files for bankruptcy protection. Private equity is a short-term investment. The goal is to exit the acquired company within three to five years either through an initial public offering or by selling to another private equity company, referred to as a secondary buyout, at a far higher price than was paid to acquire it. The business model is a little like that of house flipping: take over a company, steer it through a transition of rapid performance improvement, increase earnings, sell at a profit.

Doug Henwood and Liza Featherstone, writing in the progressive monthly magazine *In These Times* in 2018, described the process more bluntly: "The business model typically works like this: Buy a company, load it up with debt to pay yourself dividends and fees, then squeeze labor with pay cuts, layoffs and work speedup in order to cover the interest and principal payments. Investors get rich and workers get nothing."[4]

Eileen Appelbaum, an economist and the codirector of the Center for Economic and Policy Research, a Washington, DC, economic policy think tank, and Rosemary Batt, a management and labor-relations expert at Cornell University, are coauthors of *Private Equity at Work: When Wall Street Manages Main Street*. It's a foundational work, considered to be the first comprehensive examination of private equity's role in the American economy.

Appelbaum and Batt see private equity as representing "a fundamental shift in the concept of the American corporation, from a view of it as a productive enterprise and stable institution serving the needs of a broad spectrum of stakeholders to a view of it as a bundle of assets to be bought and sold with the goal of maximizing shareholder value."[5] The exclusive focus on shareholder value as the measure of the success of the corporation emerged with the decline of managerial capitalism.

The managerial model of capitalism prevailed from the 1950s to the 1970s and was based on the separation of ownership and management. The purpose of the corporation was to provide employment and benefit society through the production of consumer goods or the provision of services. Managers were the principals of power. Shareholders had little influence over decision-making. Managers sought to maximize corporate wealth, not shareholder wealth. Their careers and identities were linked to organizational success. This separation of ownership and control gave managers control over the accumulation of capital and the ability to use earnings for discretionary investments in technology, employee skills, or organizational expansion. They created job ladders that provided professional development, income growth, status, and job satisfaction that led to long organizational careers and loyal workforces. As Appelbaum and Batt phrase it, "Wall Street was at the service of Main Street."[6]

The economic recession of the 1970s—with stagnant economic growth, high inflation, and rising unemployment—led to shareholder dissatisfaction and a critique of corporate managers and the managerial model. It led to "agency theory."[7] Agency theory sees shareholders as the "principals" and residual claimants of the corporation. A residual claimant is defined as the one who has the sole claim to an organization's net cash flow. The corporate managers now become "agents" who act on behalf of the share-holders to maximize their profits. In Appelbaum and Batt's words, "Maximizing shareholder value is the exclusive goal of the corporation. Managers should return free cash flow to shareholders and use debt to finance new investment."[8] Wealth is extracted, not reinvested.

Agency theory led to the movement that replaced corporate managers with investor managers. The era of the separation of ownership and management was over. Decision-making is taken out of the hands of executives. Private equity is a hands-on investment, ownership with control. Appelbaum and Batt observe, "The law treats PE partners as investors, even though they behave as managers of the companies they buy and as employers of the people who work in those companies. Private equity funds both own and take control of companies, appoint boards of directors, hire and fire top executives, and set the direction of business strategy and employment policies."[9] Private equity companies hold formal and informal meetings and replace poorly performing management teams. The private equity firm works with the CEO of the acquired company to come up with a plan for how they will meet performance goals set by the private equity firm. Those CEOs who either can't or won't meet the private equity firm's expectations are quickly replaced with a CEO willing to follow the private equity firm's strategy. A 2018 survey found that 58% of private equity CEOs are replaced within two years of an investment. Over the lifetime of the private equity firm's ownership, CEO turnover is 73%.[10]

"Operational engineering" refers to the practice of private equity firms using their financial acumen, administrative skills, and general know-how to add value to their investments. They claim to increase profits by improving the efficiency, operations, and business strategy of the companies they acquire. Some private equity firms actually do this, adding value to the companies they acquire through the development and implementation of a business strategy or through improvements in operations that increase earnings and profit margins—for example, better supply chain management, new retail channels, or creative marketing.

In practice, private equity makes sweeping changes to cut costs and boost profits, including layoffs, pay freezes, and store closures. All too often the profits that accrue to private equity firms come not from genuinely improving the management or performance of the portfolio company but through financial engineering strategies that extract wealth without increasing the value of the portfolio company. These practices—fees, dividend recapitalization, the sale of assets, strategic bankruptcies, tax arbitrage, breach of trust—can cause long-term damage to workers, customers, vendors, and the community.

Portfolio companies pay "advisory fees" and "transaction fees" to the private equity company. Transaction fees apply to the acquisition of another company, the selling of a division of the portfolio company, or the refinancing of the portfolio company's debt. The limited partners and the general partners have a contractual agreement called the limited partner agreement. The agreement requires limited partners to pay an annual management fee of 2% of the value of the investment fund. Over a five-year period, the general partners would receive 10% of the value of the fund as a management fee regardless of how the fund performs. It is a lucrative arrangement for the private equity firm. Americans for Financial Reform, a consumer advocacy group, estimates that in 2018 investors paid $117 billion in management fees to private equity firms. Private equity firms will extract value from a company even when it is in distress. In 1997, Bain Capital acquired a majority stake in Cambridge Industries, a Michigan-based automotive plastics supplier. Although Cambridge was in serious financial trouble, having lost money for three years and accumulated significant debt, Bain continued to collect $1 million a year in "advisory" fees. From 1995 to 2000, Bain collected over $10 million in fees. In 2000, Bain took Cambridge into bankruptcy. It was bought out of bankruptcy by Meridian Automotive Systems, which eliminated more than 1,000 jobs.[11]

A dividend recapitalization is a transaction in which the private equity company borrows money, taking on new debt, usually in the form of a bank loan, in order to pay a sum of money to shareholders. Dividend recapitalizations return much—or even all—of the initial equity investment to investors. Private equity owners, uncertain of a profitable exit from a portfolio investment, resort to dividend recapitalizations to recoup their investments. Dividend recapitalizations load the acquired company with more debt and can lead to layoffs, cuts in worker pay and benefits, and bankruptcies.

In 2000, the restaurant chain Buffets, which operated 600 restaurants and employed 36,000 workers, was bought by the private equity firms Caxton-Iseman and Sentinel Capital Partners. The purchase price was $643 million. The private equity investors put up $130 million in equity. The remaining amount was debt. In June 2002, the private equity investors took $150 million in dividend recapitalization and distributed it among themselves. Over the years, the private equity firm took a total of $250 million in dividend recapitalizations. In 2008, Buffets was taken into bankruptcy. Private equity companies have been sued by creditors for driving companies into bankruptcy by dividend recapitalization. Creditors of the bankrupt Buffets sued Caxton-Iseman and charged that the dividend recapitalizations and annual service fees had drained millions of dollars from the chain and led to the 2008 bankruptcy. In September 2010, the private equity investors settled the case for more than $23 million.[12]

Private equity firms will sell off assets of the portfolio companies—"monetize" in Wall Street language—to recoup all or part of their initial equity investment. The Jones Group was a leading global designer, marketer, and wholesaler of over 35 brands in apparel, footwear, jeanswear, jewelry, and handbags, such as Nine West, Gloria Vanderbilt, and Jessica Simpson. In 2014 the private equity firm Sycamore bought the company for $1.2 billion, loading it with debt to finance the deal. The firm split it into pieces and sold off four Jones brands—Jones New York, Stuart Weitzman, Kurt Geiger, and Easy Spirit.[13] When Sycamore bought the midmarket women's clothier Talbot's, it sold "the company's credit card receivables: that is, its promise of future payments. It made over half a billion dollars for itself."[14] The most lucrative asset to sell is the portfolio company's real estate. Such practices follow what is referred to as the OpCo/PropCo model. The private equity firm will separate the real estate from the business by dividing the portfolio company into two companies: the operating company (OpCo) and the property company (PropCo). After holding the real estate long enough to qualify for favorable capital gains treatment, the private equity firm sells the property company, usually to a real estate investment trust, with the proceeds going to the private equity investors. "The new owners now require the operating company to sign long-term leases and lease the property and facilities that it previously owned from the property company—at market and sometimes above-market rents."[15] The strategy is widely used by private equity firms in industries like retail, restaurants, and nursing homes that own valuable real estate. Monetizing and divesting assets enriches the private equity firm but undermines the financial stability of the portfolio company and deprives it of an asset to weather economically difficult times.

ShopKo was a chain of department stores based in Green Bay, Wisconsin. Stores were typically placed in small to midsize communities. The company was founded in 1962 by James Ruben as ShopKo Corporation. It had slogans like, "Say hello to a good buy at ShopKo." By the end of 2005, it had more than 350 stores in

24 states. ShopKo was publicly traded on the New York Stock Exchange from 1991 until December 2005, when Sun Capital Partners took it private in an LBO for $1.1 billion. Sun Capital then sold off ShopKo's real estate for $815 million and forced the chain to lease back its formerly owned real estate. The added rent costs helped drive the store into liquidation.[16] On January 16, 2019, citing assets of less than $1 billion and $10 billion in debt, ShopKo filed for Chapter 11 bankruptcy. The bankruptcy resulted in the closure of 360 stores and the destruction of nearly 23,000 jobs.

"Tax arbitrage" refers to a strategy where individuals or corporations exploit and profit from the ways capital gains, income, and financial transactions are treated for tax purposes. Private equity's attraction to debt stems from the fact that interest on debt is tax deductible. Lower taxes increase the total value of the portfolio company by 4%–40% without an increase in economic wealth or improvements to the company. This immediately increases earnings and return to shareholders. It is essentially a transfer of wealth from taxpayers to private equity firms and their investors.

Private equity firms charge 20% of any asset appreciation. The share of profits that goes to the general partners of the private equity firm is called "carried interest." "The term 'carried interest' can be traced back to the 16th century, when trans-oceanic ship captains would frequently take a 20 percent 'interest' of whatever profits were realized from the cargo they 'carried.'" Considered to be a tax avoidance scheme, it is the most lucrative source of revenue for the general partners because of its favorable tax treatment. "Under current tax law, the carried interest paid to fund managers is taxed as if it were a profit from a long-term investment rather than what it is: compensation for performing services (managing other people's money)." This enables the general partners to pay the 20% capital gains tax rather than the 37% personal income tax. In 2021, the marginal tax rate for most American families was 22%. "This means that private equity managers pay a lower marginal tax rate on the carried interest income than most nurses, teachers, and firefighters pay on their salaries."[17]

The Pension Benefit Guaranty Corporation (PBGC) is a US federal corporation created by the Employee Retirement Income Security Act of 1974. The PBGC insures and guarantees private-sector workers' pensions. If a company goes bankrupt and its pension plan is insured by the PBGC, the PBGC will assume responsibility for continuation of pension benefits. The maximum guaranteed benefit is set by the Employee Retirement Income Security Act of 1974. Those guarantees typically range from 20% to 90% of plan benefits, according to the Society of Actuaries. The maximum guaranteed benefit is $4,500 per month.

Private equity companies use bankruptcy to reduce debt, abrogate contracts with unions and suppliers, and shed pension responsibilities. A private equity firm will take a portfolio company into bankruptcy and then buy it out of bankruptcy. The private equity firm is still the owner, but the debts of the company have been slashed and its pension liabilities have been transferred to the PBGC. The private equity firm gains by shedding obligations, but bankruptcies cost workers their jobs, benefits, severance payments, and retirement security.

According to PBGC data, from 2001 to 2014, at least 51 private equity–owned companies rid themselves of pension plans by bankruptcy, dumping $1.6 billion in obligations onto the PBGC and costing over 100,000 affected workers and retirees at least $128 million.[18] Included in that number were well-known companies such as Hostess, Friendly's restaurants, the auto parts maker Delphi, and the retailer Eddie Bauer. The number of bankruptcies strained the resources at the PBGC and raised the specter of a taxpayer bailout.

Friendly's Ice Cream Corporation was started as an ice cream parlor selling double-dip cones in Springfield, Massachusetts, by brothers Curtis and Prestley Blake in 1935 with a $547 loan from their parents. It grew to become a family restaurant with 515 franchised stores throughout the Northeast and several southeastern states. In addition, Friendly's 22 ice cream flavors were distributed through more than 4,000 supermarkets. In August 2007, Sun Capital took Friendly's private in an LBO for $337 million, including $175 million of long-term debt. Just four years later, in 2011, with $297 million in debt, Sun Capital took Friendly's into bankruptcy. Immediately after Friendly's closed 65 stores, laid off 1,260 workers, and sought Chapter 11 bankruptcy protection, another Sun Capital unit moved to acquire the restaurant chain. A third Sun Capital affiliate offered a loan to finance the chain's operations while the company was in bankruptcy. In December 2011, Sun Capital was able to "buy" Friendly's in an auction using a practice called credit bidding. A secured creditor is a lender whose loan is backed by collateral. If the borrower defaults on the loan, the lender can sell the collateral to regain some of the money lost. In a bankruptcy case, a secured creditor has certain privileges that unsecured creditors don't have. Credit bidding is a section of the Bankruptcy Code that allows a secured creditor to obtain possession of a bankrupt company at auction simply by agreeing to forgive the debt that the company owes rather than paying cash for the company. It frees the buyer from any liability to other creditors, including vendors, pension plans, and other unsecured creditors. Sun Capital was able to retain ownership of Friendly's, the $75 million loan that another Sun affiliate had made to see the restaurant chain through the bankruptcy period was forgiven, and the restructuring shifted liability for Friendly's pension plan to the federal government's PBGC so Sun Capital no longer was responsible for the chain's $115 million in pension obligations to its nearly 6,000 employees and retirees.[19]

Breach of trust occurs when private equity firms fail to honor formal and implicit contracts and understandings with stakeholders like vendors. In an article, "The 6 Things a Private Equity Firm Will Do after It Buys Your Business," Jim Schleckser writes that private equity firms will try to increase cash flow by "stretching out the terms with your suppliers. If you have built up loyal relationships with your suppliers where you pay them every 30 days, expect them to now get pushed out to 45 or even 60 days before they get paid. The PE firms will also move aggressively to reduce any inventory you have on hand."[20] Steward Health Care owns nine hospitals, rehabs, and health-care facilities in eastern Massachusetts in mostly working-class, low-income towns. Several lawsuits alleged that Steward had not paid vendors for supplies and services in months, totaling over $7.5 million. The vendors included providers of computer software, security guards, cleaning services, and electrical wiring. Steward was sued by two advertising firms for more than $2 million; a linen services provider for $317,000 in delinquent payments; and a New York utility firm for $250,000 in natural gas bills. The restaurant Cape Cod Cafe stopped delivering pizzas to Good Samaritan Medical Center in Brockton because Steward hadn't paid until six months had passed and thousands of dollars in bills had piled up.[21] Private equity firms will terminate contracts altogether. The country's second-largest private equity–owned dermatology practice, U.S. Dermatology Partners, changed vendors to a cheaper brand of needles and sutures of such poor quality they would often break off in a patient's wound and have to be removed.[22]

The private equity strategy is "buy and build," to expand by acquisitions. Increasing the size increases the value of the company and the likelihood of a more financially prosperous exit. The strategy also gives it what is known as economies of scale. The increased size of a business—scale—gives the private equity firm economic advantages such as greater purchasing power through the bulk buying of materials and the ability to renegotiate contracts with vendors on supplies and equipment, get lower interest rates on bank loans, streamline administrative staff, and lay off employees who are no longer needed. The private equity business model is to take on increasing amounts of debt to finance LBOs and to grow through "add-ons." In health care, firms begin by acquiring a small hospital system, called a platform company, in an LBO. They use that company to add smaller hospitals in geographically dispersed regions, creating a national, multistate hospital system. The median deal size of LBOs in health care is in the range of $60–$70 million, an amount too small to come under the jurisdiction and scrutiny of the Federal Trade Commission and antitrust regulators. By making a series of small deals, private equity–owned hospital systems can build medical empires, what health economist Thomas Wollmann terms "stealth consolidation."[23]

Private equity companies are attracted not to random companies but to industries. They look for specific industries for various reasons such as sufficient cash flow or valuable real estate. Over the last decade, private equity has decimated several industries, leaving behind swaths of destruction that have changed the landscape of American life. Bankruptcies have deep and long-lasting effects. Wide-scale job losses devastate working families, have far-ranging impacts on local economies and small businesses, and ultimately ripple throughout the national economy as suppliers feel the downstream effects. In July 2018, just months after Toys "R" Us shut down, Mattel, the maker of Barbie and Hot Wheels, announced it was laying off 2,200 workers after its sales dropped by 14%. According to Moody's Investors Service, Toys "R" Us was the third-largest taxpayer in Wayne, New Jersey, and its $2.1 million payment in fiscal year 2016 was 2.5% of its operating revenue.[24] The disappearance of so many independent, small to midsize businesses has led to the growth and concentration of retailers like Amazon, Walmart, and Target, which have grown bigger, more profitable, and more powerful. In 2016, the four largest US retailers earned 90% of total profits.

In "Private Equity Pillage: Grocery Stores and Workers at Risk," Appelbaum and Batt describe the effect of private equity on the grocery store industry. Grocery chains employ 2.8 million workers in small towns and cities throughout America. They're vital to the economics and the sense of community in the neighborhoods and towns they serve. Between 2015 and 2018, seven large regional grocery chains filed for bankruptcy. All were owned by private equity. The job loss was staggering. The bankrupted private equity-owned grocery chains included A&P, once the largest grocery store in America with 296 stores and 285,000 employees; Southeastern Grocers, with over 730 stores and over 50,000 employees; and Marsh Supermarkets, with 116 stores and 14,000 employees. In the seven bankruptcies, tens of thousands of workers lost their jobs and saw reduced pensions. This carnage concentrated the industry. Today, in over 200 regions of the country, Walmart is responsible for 50% or more of all grocery sales.[25]

The media blamed low-cost competitors like Walmart and high-end markets like Whole Foods, which was acquired by Amazon for $13.7 billion in 2017. But the real culprits were the private equity owners who extracted millions from the grocery stores in fees, dividend recapitalizations, and stripped assets that could have been invested in upgrading stores, improving products and services, training employees, and increasing wages. Debt burdened, financially unstable, paying rent on property they once owned, these grocery chains lost the ability and resources to compete in a changing market.

Private equity is attracted to retail because of its stable cash flow and lucrative real estate portfolio. The history of private equity and retail is one of bankruptcies that have seen the disappearance of iconic stores in the United States. Between 2008 and

2011, 260 private equity–owned companies filed for bankruptcy, including Linen 'n Things, Fortunoff Fine Jewelry and Silverware, Sharper Image, the online retailer Lillian Vernon, *Reader's Digest*, and Mervyn's Department Store, which had 257 stores and 30,000 employees. The year 2017 is known as the year of the "retail apocalypse" when seven major US chains went bankrupt. Among them were household names such as Toys "R" Us, Payless, the Limited, H. H. Gregg, and True Religion. What they had in common was that private equity firms had loaded the companies with unsustainable debt. Jim Baker, Maggie Corser, and Eli Vitulli, in a July 2019 report titled *Pirate Equity*, said that between 2012 and 2019, a total of 1.3 million people lost their jobs in private equity retail chain bankruptcies. The authors noted that Wall Street firms had destroyed eight times as many retail jobs as they had created in the past decade. In the first three months of 2019, private equity–owned retailers closed 4,680 stores of name brands like Barneys New York, Sugarfina, Sears, K-Mart, Charlotte Russe, Gymboree, Sports Authority, and RadioShack. Private equity–owned retailers that filed for bankruptcy in 2020 include J. C. Penney, Circuit City, Neiman Marcus, J. Crew, True Religion, Lucky Brand, and Sur La Table.[26]

In April 1948, during the postwar baby boom, Charles Philip Lazarus began selling cradles and cribs from his father's bicycle store. He soon opened his first store, Children's Bargain Town, a children's furniture store, in the Adams Morgan neighborhood of Washington, DC, focusing primarily on strollers and baby cribs. In June 1957, Lazarus opened the first Toys "R" Us, dedicated exclusively to toys rather than furniture, in Rockville, Maryland. Lazarus also designed and stylized the Toys "R" Us logo, which featured a backward *R* as if a small child had written it.

Toys "R" Us eventually grew to over 1,600 stores worldwide. In July 2001, it opened a flagship store on Broadway in New York's Times Square. The 110,000-square-foot store, the largest in the world, included a Barbie zone with a life-size dreamhouse, a Jurassic Park–themed area with a lifelike T-Rex, and a working Ferris wheel that was 60 feet high.

On March 17, 2005, the private equity firms Bain Capital Partners, KKR, and Vornado Realty Trust took ownership of Toy "R" Us in a $6.6 billion LBO. The transaction loaded $5.3 billion of debt onto the company, requiring almost $400 million in interest payments annually, on top of management and advisory fees. The debt was insurmountable. On September 18, 2017, unable to innovate, and after refinancing several times, cutting staff, and underinvesting in stores, Toys "R" Us filed for Chapter 11 bankruptcy. Most of its $5 billion debt had not been paid down since the buyout 12 years earlier. The company had not had an annual profit since 2013.[27]

The Toys "R" Us liquidation sales began on March 23, 2018. On June 29, 2018, after 70 years of operations, Toys "R" Us permanently closed all 735 of its remaining US stores. Over 33,000 employees lost their jobs. Many former Toys "R" Us employees were nearing retirement when the business closed. They lost their pensions as well as vacation and sick pay they were owed. None of them were offered severance payments. Vendors lost $350 million. Executives fared better. Informed by the company's lawyers that executive bonuses would not be approved once the company filed for bankruptcy, CEO David Brandon ordered bonuses of $2.8 million to himself and other top executives three days before the bankruptcy filing.[28] After months of protest, two of the investors—Bain and KKR—gave $10 million each to an employee severance fund, less than the $75 million the attorney for the employees estimated would cover full severance. Vornado Realty Trust did not join the fund. A lawsuit from creditors that lost hundreds of millions of dollars in the Toys "R" Us bankruptcy alleged that between 2014 and 2017, years in which Toys "R" Us made no profit, $18 million in fees was paid to Bain Capital, KKR, and Vornado

Realty Trust. At a 2019 hearing titled "America for Sale? An Examination of the Practices of Private Funds," Giovanna De La Rosa, who had worked at Toys "R" Us for 20 years, told lawmakers, "Toys 'R' Us had a decades-long severance policy—a week of pay for every year of service to the company. But when our company liquidated, the employees were left with nothing. . . . My coworkers and I were left with nothing while the executives and private equity owners walked away with millions."[29]

In a 2018 report for the Institute for New Economic Thinking, Appelbaum and Batt wrote about private equity's increasing presence in the health-care industry. "'It's been an ongoing interest of ours because we felt that it was the worst sector private equity could be involved in,' Batt said. The stakes were higher than in toy retailing: health care was a complex and heavily regulated industry, and drastic cost reductions had the potential to affect people's safety."[30]

In her 2019 essay "How Private Equity Makes You Sicker," Appelbaum describes the closure of Hahnemann University Hospital as "one of the more egregious cases of private equity wealth extraction."[31]

Center City comprises the central business district and central neighborhoods of Philadelphia. It is the most densely populated downtown area in the United States, after Midtown Manhattan. Hahnemann University Hospital was a 496-bed Level 1 trauma center in Center City and the teaching hospital of Drexel University College of Medicine. It was founded in 1848 and named for Samuel Hahnemann, the founder of homeopathy, and was the first homeopathic medical college in the United States. Grace Kelly was born at Hahnemann on November 12, 1929. Considered a safety net hospital, Hahnemann had been serving the poor of Philadelphia for more than 170 years. It was also affiliated with St. Christopher's Hospital for Children in North Philadelphia.

On January 12, 2018, Dallas-based Tenet Healthcare sold Hahnemann and St. Christopher's to the California private equity firm

Paladin Healthcare in partnership with Chicago-based health-care real estate private equity firm Harrison Street Real Estate Capital for $170 million. Paladin was owned by investment banker Joel Freedman. After the purchase, it was renamed the American Academic Health System (AAHS). The deal was financed with at least $35 million in debt provided by Apollo Global Management, one of the largest private equity firms in the country, which later loaned Paladin another $20 million.

The year following the sale was one of turmoil. Hahnemann saw five CEOs come and go. The Pennsylvania Association of Staff Nurses and Allied Professionals, representing 850 nurses at Hahnemann, was unable to agree on the terms for a new contract with AAHS, claiming unsafe staffing was jeopardizing patient safety. On January 4, 2019, Hahnemann cut 30 management positions and closed three primary care offices. In April, Hahnemann laid off 175 employees, citing declining revenue and fewer patients. The layoffs included 65 nurses, 22 service and technical workers, and 88 nonunion employees.

On June 26, AAHS announced that, because of unsustainable financial losses, Hahnemann Hospital would close in September. On June 30, Freedman announced that he had filed for Chapter 11 bankruptcy and immediate liquidation of his assets. The union made appeals to Philadelphia mayor Jim Kenney, the Philadelphia City Council, the Pennsylvania legislature, and Pennsylvania governor Tom Wolf to prevent the closure of the hospital, but to no avail.

Once AAHS announced plans to close the hospital, numerous efforts were made to prevent it. Drexel University filed an unsuccessful lawsuit, claiming that it would be a violation of the academic agreement between the university and the hospital. On June 27, the Pennsylvania secretary of health, Rachel Levine, wrote to AAHS leadership ordering a "cease and desist" of any action toward hospital closure without a state-approved plan. In the "cease and desist" letter, Levine had concluded that an immediate closure of Hahnemann or the termination of any services could cause irreparable harm to the health and safety of patients in Philadelphia, especially during the Fourth of July holiday week. Despite this, AAHS began cutting vital hospital services, including trauma and cardiothoracic surgery services, within days of the closure announcement.

On June 29, Hahnemann withdrew its Level 1 trauma designation. On July 10, Hahnemann was ordered by a Philadelphia County Court of Common Pleas judge to keep the Center City hospital open until the Philadelphia Health Department approved a closure plan. On July 12, the hospital announced it would halt all nonemergency surgeries and procedures and would stop delivering babies. On Tuesday, July 16, Hahnemann announced it would close its maternity unit on the coming Friday. The Drexel University College of Medicine's department of obstetrics and gynecology was forced to send letters to patients informing them they would need to find someplace else to deliver their babies. On July 17, the hospital stopped admissions. It discharged its last inpatient on July 26. On August 16, it closed its emergency room.

Hahnemann's closure also meant that 550 medical residents in over 30 specialties were compelled to find new placements to continue their graduate medical education. In a repudiation of the mission of academic medicine, Hahnemann saw the residents as an asset to be monetized for profit and made the decision to auction the residency positions.

A consortium of Northeast hospitals bid $55 million for the positions. The Centers for Medicare and Medicaid Services (CMS), which pays hospitals roughly $100,000 annually per resident slot, considered the sale of the residency programs illegal and filed court documents objecting to it. CMS argued that the auction could set a dangerous precedent, particularly for struggling hospitals, to use resident physician positions as valuable assets to be sold. In a statement, House Energy and Commerce Committee chairman Frank Pallone Jr. said the approval of the $55 million sale would send a signal to Wall Street that there is money to be made off the downfall of community hospitals.

The sale was also opposed by the State of Pennsylvania, the Accreditation Council for Graduate Medical Education, the Association of American Medical Colleges, the Pennsylvania Association of Staff Nurses and Allied Professionals, and the Educational Commission for Foreign Medical Graduates, which sponsors the J-1 visas for international doctors in training.

On September 5, in a defeat for the federal government, US bankruptcy judge Kevin Gross ruled that Freedman could sell Hahnemann's medical residency program to a consortium of six local health systems led by Thomas Jefferson University Hospital.[32] The ruling came just one day before Hahnemann had pledged to close its doors forever.

Hahnemann was a cluster of seven medical buildings and a parking garage on a nearly six-acre square block between Broad Street and 15th Street and between Race Street and Vine Street. It was at the northern end of what's known as the Avenue of the Arts, a gentrified neighborhood of theaters, music venues, a major entertainment center, restaurants, and the University of the Arts, and cater-corner to the Pennsylvania Convention Center. A CNN report described the area as ideal for high-end retail stores and luxury condominiums.[33]

When Hahnemann was sold, the hospital real estate, estimated at $58 million, was separated from the operating business and was excluded from the bankruptcy filing. It was widely believed that Freedman's scheme all along was to drive the hospital into bankruptcy, liquidate the assets, and sell the lucrative real estate.

On July 30, 2020, a year after Hahnemann filed for bankruptcy, Natalie Kostelni wrote in the *Philadelphia Business Journal* that the real estate once occupied by Hahnemann University Hospital in

Philadelphia had come up for sale. She described the site as something rare in a dense urban setting: a contiguous stretch of buildings and land with upwards of 3 million square feet for potentially new development in a highly visible area of Center City. She called it a generational development opportunity.[34]

4

Ardent, 2001–2020

"The first Sisters of Charity arrived in New Mexico Territory in 1865 from Cincinnati at the request of Bishop Lamy [the first archbishop of Santa Fe] with the mission of serving all people regardless of race, religion or ability to pay. Hundreds of sisters followed."[1] They would make a lasting impact on the state's education and health-care systems, establishing schools and hospitals such as the St. Vincent Hospital and Orphanage and the St. Elizabeth Shelter for the Homeless in Santa Fe. "The Sisters of Charity opened the first nursing school, the first schools for X-ray and laboratory technicians, and the first blood bank in New Mexico."[2] In 1889, the Jesuits, who had been teaching in Albuquerque since 1875, offered the Sisters of Charity land east of the city to build a hospital. In 1900 Sister Blandina Seagle, who had cofounded public and Catholic schools in Santa Fe, returned to Albuquerque for two years to help start St. Joseph Hospital. Construction on the land was started in 1901.[3] Albuquerque's first hospital, opened by the Sisters of Charity in 1902, was St. Joseph Hospital and Sanatorium. It had 95 beds with a 40-bed annex for tuberculosis patients.

Sister Zita Denman served as the first administrator of the hospital.[4]

In 1927, when Albuquerque's population reached 35,000, the sisters began building a new hospital to accommodate the growth. The 152-bed hospital opened in 1930. In 1954 the Sisters of Charity closed St. Joseph Sanatorium, and it became a convent. By 1966, Albuquerque's population had grown to 275,000. The sisters demolished the former sanatorium and broke ground for a new hospital. St. Joseph Medical Center, "a 12-story, $10.8 million facility opened in 1968, with 349 beds, a neurology department, rehabilitation department, pediatrics department and youth care center."[5] In 1984, it added St. Joseph West Mesa Hospital and, a year later, St. Joseph Northeast Heights Medical Center. In 1988 the St. Joseph Rehabilitation Hospital and Outpatient Center was added.

In 1996, the Sisters of Charity joined with two other national health-care systems, Catholic Health Corporation and Franciscan Health System, to form Catholic Health Initiatives (CHI), a nonprofit, faith-based health system. Their goal: to develop a national health ministry overseen by a religious-lay partnership that would strengthen community health care.

During the five and a half years it owned the system, CHI, which operated 63 hospitals and 44 long-term care facilities in 19 states, invested $50 million in the St. Joseph system. It demurred on investing another $35 million that St. Joseph needed and put St. Joseph up for sale in November 2001. CHI expressed its desire to sell St. Joseph to another Catholic health-care organization or to another nonprofit provider.

Nashville-based Behavioral Healthcare Corporation was founded in 1993 by Charles A. Elcan. It operated behavioral health facilities and psychiatric hospitals in Tulsa, Oklahoma, and Amarillo, Texas. In May 2001, Welsh, Carson, Anderson, and Stowe, a private equity firm based in New York, bought the company for $145 million and changed its name to Ardent.

In March 2002, Ardent bought the St. Joseph system from CHI. That system now included three acute care hospitals, a rehabilitation hospital, a health maintenance organization, physician practices, and partial ownership of several other businesses. The sale meant that St. Joseph went from a nonprofit to a for-profit. Ardent at that time owned 24 hospitals in 12 states and had 4,400 employees.

In July 2002, Ardent announced it was buying the Lovelace Health System from Cigna Corporation for $211 million. The purchase included the 225-bed Lovelace Hospital and the Lovelace Health Plan. Ardent merged the two systems and formed Lovelace Sandia Health System. Sandia now had five hospitals, including its main hospital on Gibson Boulevard; a multispecialty physician group practice; the Lovelace Health Plan and MedicarePlus Health Plan; S.E.D. Medical Laboratories; and 15 primary care centers. The purchases gave Ardent control of about 40% of Albuquerque's hospital beds.

From 2001 to 2004, Ardent, following the private equity business model, acquired nine small hospitals and clinics in the Southeast and Southwest. It did so by taking on debt. In 2001, Ardent received $2 million of development capital from Clayton Associates and, in 2003, $4.58 million of development capital from Peloton Equity. Ardent also took on an undisclosed amount of debt in the form of a loan.[6]

On May 11, 2004, Ardent announced that it had reached an agreement to purchase the Hillcrest HealthCare System of Tulsa, Oklahoma, for $281.2 million. The Hillcrest system included 6,000 employees, 1,800 physicians, 39 facilities, 6 metropolitan Tulsa hospitals, 10 regional hospitals throughout eastern Oklahoma, and 2 long-term care facilities. It also included two tertiary hospitals, both located in Tulsa—the 557-bed Hillcrest Medical Center and the 331-bed Tulsa Regional Medical Center, which is also the nation's largest osteopathic teaching hospital.[7]

On March 10, 2005, Ardent completed its move to acute care when it announced it would be selling 20 inpatient psychiatric facilities to Psychiatric Solutions for $560 million. It changed its name to Ardent Health Services.

On January 5, 2006, Winthrop Quigley, in the *Albuquerque Journal*, reflected on Ardent's conflict-laden entry into Albuquerque's health-care market: "the physician alienation, the employee complaints, the resignations and ousters, the financial problems, and the bad press."[8] The bad press included a March 28, 2005, article in the *Albuquerque Business Journal* that reported the Albuquerque Regional Medical Center, part of Ardent's Lovelace Sandia Health System, was facing an investigation by the New Mexico Department of Health after a preliminary probe found a number of deficiencies: a pathology specimen was mislabeled; a patient received a blood transfusion even though it conflicted with the patient's religious beliefs; a patient was operated on with nonsterilized equipment and subsequently required six weeks of intravenous antibiotics; a patient needed to return to surgery because doctors had left a surgical sponge in the patient's body. The investigation not only revealed a breakdown in quality control, it also found that the hospital did not have a quality assurance program to assess and improve its performance in patient care. A March 11, 2005, letter to the hospital from the Centers for Medicare and Medicaid Services stated, "These deficiencies have been determined to be of such a serious nature as to substantially limit your hospital's capacity to render adequate care and prevent it from being in compliance with all the Conditions of Participation for Hospitals," and warned about a potential fund cutoff by the Centers for Medicare and Medicaid Services. The letter also noted that all 17 hospital doctors who were interviewed during the investigation said that they "were extremely concerned about the reduced staffing in the nursing department and the lack of permanent, well-trained nursing staff for the past two years."[9]

In 2006, Lovelace Sandia closed the Lovelace Medical Center on Gibson. Lovelace Medical Center and St. Joseph's Hospital were consolidated into a single facility on St. Joseph's downtown campus. The 263-bed hospital was now known as Lovelace Medical Center. The 559,000-square-foot Gibson hospital was decommissioned and put up for sale. Northeast Heights Medical Center became Lovelace Women's Hospital.

The Lovelace Medical Group maintained an outpatient behavioral health clinic in the Journal Center, a business and residential community in northwest Albuquerque, that served 6,700 patients. Lovelace Sandia announced that "Lovelace's regular outpatient behavioral health care will be discontinued effective May 30, 2006."[10] No reason was given for the closure, but behavioral health is not considered a profitable specialty: "Profitable specialties," Quigley writes, "like cardiology, subsidized money-losers, like behavioral health."[11] The announcement jeopardized the continuity of care of thousands of New Mexicans. Local organizations interceded to mitigate the impact of the closure. To ensure patients received the care they needed, the Bernalillo County Local Collaborative worked with Lovelace "to extend the transition period for patients to receive discharge counseling and transition assistance through the end of June."[12] A transition team from ValueOptions New Mexico was working closely with Lovelace to reach behavioral health consumers who were receiving publicly funded care. "As the statewide entity for publicly-funded behavioral health services, we want to ensure that no disruptions in service occur while Lovelace Medical Group ends its outpatient behavioral health care," said Pam Galbraith, CEO of ValueOptions New Mexico.[13] Lovelace was closing the clinic, but it wanted the practitioners who cared "for those patients to end their employment with Lovelace and set up their own practice, with Lovelace's help. These new private-practice physicians would take care of the same patients they had been seeing today as Lovelace employees."[14]

"Regardless of the staff's decision," Quigley writes, "the clinic would close. Employees and patients who contacted the *Journal* said they didn't like the plan and were suspicious of the company's motives and competence."[15]

In 2007, Lovelace's 225-physician medical group, the heart of the old Lovelace system, announced it would end its relationship with Ardent and enter into private practice. Negotiations for Lovelace Medical Group to spin off from Lovelace had begun in 2005. CEO Harry Magnes said morale among the doctors was low and that one in five doctors was leaving each year. The final decision came after Ardent laid off 100 employees and divided the organization into three subsidiaries—health plan, hospital, and medical group—that no longer shared profits from ancillary services. Ancillary services such as imaging, ultrasound, laboratory, pathology, and radiology are highly profitable. The revenue was vital to the success of Lovelace Medical Group. After Ardent broke up the old Lovelace structure, it took over ancillary services, and none of the ancillary revenue was distributed to the physician group. As a result, the medical group began to lose money.[16] Economists make a distinction between profit seeking and rent seeking in private equity–owned companies. Profit seeking creates new wealth through innovation and growth. Rent seeking doesn't create wealth; it manipulates resources and redistributes wealth to the private equity company.

Ardent's depreciation of the physician group was a direct contrast to the historical role of physicians in the Lovelace system. Under David J. Ottensmeyer's leadership, the medical staff was integrated centrally in the operation. Physicians had representation on the executive committee of the organization and on the clinic's board of governors. Ottensmeyer believed if the staff's doctors were to have managerial authority, they should be prepared through formal study of modern management and health-care administration. During the 1980s, the Lovelace Medical Center became a national leader in the high standards of training it required for its modern physician-managers.

Richard Rolston was a pediatrician with Lovelace Medical Group for 11 years. He was also the CEO of Lovelace Medical Center and the Lovelace Medical Group until he resigned in 2005. "I have great respect for Lovelace and the people there," Rolston said. "The reason the group is choosing to do this is because Ardent took it down a path that has devastated the group. Lovelace is trying to get back to where they were before and to regain the trust of the community."[17]

The desire to return to founding principles was echoed by Magnes: "This gives us an opportunity to get back to our roots in patient care, research, and education. It allows us to partner with Lovelace, but bring decision-making to physicians."[18] In 2007, Lovelace Medical Group would be resurrected as ABQ Health Partners, of which Magnes would become president and CEO.

The years between 2010 and 2017 would see Ardent continue to make financial moves, expanding through acquisitions and selling assets, but they would also see discord between Ardent and the health-care community of New Mexico: a public feud with its original physician group; conflict with neighboring hospitals; and the loss of lucrative service contracts, which weakened it financially, reduced its role in the health-care world of New Mexico, and affected the insurance coverage and access to care of thousands of New Mexicans.

Christus St. Vincent Regional Medical Center in Santa Fe had been a contracted provider of members of the Lovelace Health Plan for more than 15 years. On August 20, 2010, it severed ties with the Lovelace Health Plan. This meant that, except for emergencies, anyone on that insurance plan would not be able to get treatment from northern New Mexico's largest hospital or any of its health-care centers. The decision affected over 14,000 members. The dispute was over reimbursement. Lovelace said the decision by the hospital not to renew the contract was "unfortunate." St. Vincent spokesman Arturo Delgado countered that what was "unfortunate" was that Ardent Health, Lovelace's parent company, had attempted to "unilaterally reduce reimbursement rates, contrary to terms of the contract."[19]

In an eight-month span, Lovelace acquired two New Mexican hospitals. On May 9, 2011, Lovelace signed an agreement to purchase the Heart Hospital of New Mexico from MedCath Corporation for $119 million. On January 3, 2012, Lovelace announced that it was selling its laboratories to New Jersey–based Quest Diagnostics. Quest would acquire a 50,000-square-foot lab facility, nine patient service centers in Albuquerque and Rio Rancho, and six additional centers throughout the state. Lovelace would outsource its own labs at its four hospitals to Quest Diagnostics. On January 14, 2012, Lovelace signed a letter of intent to buy the 26-bed Roswell Regional Hospital and its Family Care Clinic.

On September 10, 2012, ABQ Health Partners announced it had merged with California-based HealthCare Partners, one of the nation's largest medical groups and physician networks. Magnes said the merger would facilitate its move from a fee-for-service model to a coordinated care model. At that time, ABQ Health Partners and Lovelace were in negotiations for a new contract. On October 9, 2012, Magnes announced that Lovelace had broken off negotiations and had notified ABQ Health Partners that it was terminating the contracts that allowed 74 ABQ Health Partners providers to treat Lovelace patients in the system's hospitals. The contracts, some of which had been in place since 2007, affected ABQ Health Partners providers in Lovelace Medical Center,

Lovelace Westside Hospital, Lovelace Women's Hospital, and Lovelace Rehabilitation Hospital. Thousands of Lovelace members had to choose whether to keep their Lovelace insurance or leave Lovelace in order to keep their ABQ Health Partners providers. Magnes contended that it was a financial decision on Lovelace's part, that Lovelace saw coordinated care as a threat to the profitability of its hospitals. He said Lovelace wanted a fee-for-service model that pays for every medical procedure performed and test ordered."[20] Coordinated care, or value-based care, is a health-care delivery model under which providers—hospitals and doctors—are paid based on the health outcomes of their patients and the quality of services rendered. It shifts the health-care system away from delivering services to delivering results. It pays health-care providers for making their patients healthier instead of paying them for how many services they provide. In addition, by promoting prevention, patients have less need for medical services such as acute care, emergency room visits, and lab testing.

The relationship between Lovelace and ABQ Health Partners became public and acrimonious. On October 22, 2012, Lovelace filed a lawsuit against ABQ Health Partners. Lovelace claimed the physician group was engaging in a "smear campaign" to steer Lovelace members to other health insurers.[21] Lovelace asked the state district court in Albuquerque to stop ABQ Health Partners from trying to get its patients to switch insurance companies. Lovelace CEO Ron Stern released a statement saying that "ABQ Health Partners had been outright instructing its patients through coercive, misleading and illegal means that the patients must join another health plan ... [and] directing patients to plans that are more financially beneficial to ABQ Health Partners."[22] ABQ Health Partners responded with a statement that, "at ABQ Health Partners, we are trying to educate our patients about their basic rights. Lovelace Health Plan is trying to prevent this through a new lawsuit and through misleading advertisements and confusing communications. It is an attempt by Lovelace Health Plan to interfere with the rights of doctors and patients to communicate with each other."[23] On November 8, 2012, the state district court denied a request by Lovelace to prevent ABQ Health Partners from communicating with its patients. The court's ruling validated ABQ Health Partners' position that the lawsuit was frivolous.

In June 2012 Cigna announced it would end its more than 20-year-old contract with Lovelace to treat its 18,000 members in the Albuquerque area. Patients would need to find new medical providers by July 1, when the contract would lapse. Cigna would contract instead with Presbyterian Healthcare Services.[24]

On October 19, 2012, in a move to rebuild its physician practice, Lovelace Health System acquired Southwest Medical Associates, a 33-year-old physician-owned, multispecialty medical practice.

Over a 10-month span, Lovelace lost or relinquished almost the entirety of its insured health plan members.

On February 4, 2013, the New Mexico Human Services Department announced that Lovelace Health Plan had lost its bid to become one of the four insurance companies to participate in New Mexico's $4 billion Medicaid program known as Centennial Care. The contracts were awarded to Blue Cross Blue Shield of New Mexico, Presbyterian Health Plan, Molina Healthcare of New Mexico, and UnitedHealthcare Community Plan of New Mexico. Lovelace appealed the decision. On May 24, 2013, New Mexico Human Services Department secretary Sidonie Squier notified the Lovelace Health Plan that its appeal had been denied. Lovelace's 84,000 Medicaid members accounted for more than a third of the health plan's revenue. Lovelace has been providing managed care to Medicaid beneficiaries since 1998.[25]

Molina Healthcare of New Mexico held "the highest NCQA [National Committee for Quality Assurance] ranking among

Medicaid plans in the state . . . [and] was one of four managed care plans awarded a contract as part of the New Mexico Human Services Department's Centennial Care program."[26] The National Committee for Quality Assurance "evaluates health plans on the quality of care patients receive, how happy patients are with their care and health plans' efforts to keep improving."[27] In July 2013, Lovelace announced it had sold its 84,000 Lovelace Health Plan Medicaid memberships to Molina for $53.5 million.

In November 2013, Lovelace agreed to sell its insurance operation to Blue Cross Blue Shield of New Mexico. The loss of 84,000 Medicaid managed care members left it with only 108,000 insured health plan members. Lovelace CEO Ron Stern said in an interview that the Lovelace Health Plan "became too small to survive" when it lost its Medicaid bid earlier that year. Lovelace had been offering insurance since 1973, when Lovelace was still a physician-owned multispecialty medical practice. When Ardent bought Lovelace in 2002, the Lovelace insurance plan had 167,700 commercial, Medicare, and Medicaid members.[28]

In a March 3, 2013, letter to a Bernalillo County commissioner and in an op-ed in the *Albuquerque Journal*, Lovelace Health System expressed its opposition to plans of the University of New Mexico to spend $146 million on a new hospital.[29] Stern wrote that Albuquerque did not need a new big hospital in the downtown area. Stern offered the University of New Mexico Hospital (UNM) a bed-sharing agreement with Lovelace Medical Center that would help alleviate the overcrowding and excessive delays in UNM's emergency department and save the taxpayers $146 million. An article two days later in the *Journal* said Lovelace's letter wasn't pure altruism; it was about business and empty hospital beds it would like to fill with paying customers. Lovelace Medical Center had a 61% occupancy rate. UNM's occupancy rate was more than 90%. Officials with UNMH contended, "The problem is bigger than just a lack of beds. It's a problem of having the right medical staff at the bedside. So even if Lovelace could offer beds, that wouldn't solve the problem of providing proper care."[30]

In March 2015, Walgreens, the Deerfield, Illinois–based drugstore chain, announced it was acquiring 11 Lovelace retail pharmacies and closing 6 of them. The pharmacies on Montgomery, Carlisle, Tramway at Encantado, Gibson, Rio Bravo, and Coors would close. Lovelace pharmacies at Journal Center, Tower at Walter Street, and Juan Tabo and one each in Santa Fe and Rio Rancho would be converted to Walgreens pharmacies.

On September 5, 2017, Lovelace Medical Group announced it would terminate its contract with Presbyterian Health Plan effective January 1. Lovelace Medical Group/Southwest Medical Associates providers would no longer accept Presbyterian insurance. Lovelace refused comment on the reasons for its decision. The decision would have affected about 7,400 customers. In its letter, Lovelace suggested patients choose a health insurance plan that Lovelace does accept. Brandon Fryar, Presbyterian Health Plan president, released a statement that Presbyterian was working with community medical providers as well as Presbyterian Medical Group to ensure the 7,400 members affected by Lovelace's decision would continue to have access to quality care.[31]

The financial crisis of 2008 delayed the plans of Welsh, Carson, Anderson, and Stowe (WCAS) to exit its investment in Ardent in the traditional three-to-five-year period. Private equity deal making collapsed. Private equity companies' value fell below or remained near their original purchase price. They were unable to exit their portfolio company investments without incurring losses or lower-than-expected returns. New private equity investments fell from $245 billion to $20 billion between the fourth quarter of 2007 and the second quarter of 2009. In 2009, 100 private equity–owned companies filed for bankruptcy protection, 69 in 2010, and 42 in 2011. The economic impact persisted until 2013. During that time, Ardent took on a significant amount of debt. In

April 2010, the company took a $475 million dividend recapitalization: investors and banks provided $395 million in loans, $75 million in revolving lines of credit, and $5 million of senior debt. Senior debt, or a senior note, is a loan that takes precedence over other debts in the event the company declares bankruptcy and is forced into liquidation. It is collateralized by assets. In 2012, Bank of America, Merrill Lynch, and Barclays led a $1.02 billion debt refinancing of Ardent's senior secured credit facilities. In finance, a "facility," whether it's called a loan facility or a credit facility, is a preapproved loan provided by the bank to a company where the company can borrow money when it needs to without having to reapply for a loan each time. In March 2013, Apollo Investment provided $20 million of debt financing in the form of a second lien-secured debt.[32]

It wasn't until 2015 that WCAS found a buyer. A real estate investment trust is a company that owns or operates income-producing real estate. The trust leases space and collects rents on the properties, then distributes that income as dividends to shareholders. Individual investors earn dividends from real estate investments without having to buy, manage, or finance any properties themselves. Ventas is a Chicago-based real estate investment trust that owns 1,200 properties such as senior living communities, nursing homes, medical office buildings, inpatient rehabilitation facilities, and long-term care centers throughout the United States and Canada with a market value of $25 billion. It owns and manages approximately 27 million square feet of medical office building space across 31 states that draws over 35 million patients each year. On August 4, 2015, Ventas announced its acquisition of Ardent Health Services for $1.75 billion. As part of the deal, Ardent Health Services would distribute about $75 million in excess cash to its shareholders. At WCAS's exit, Ardent was generating $2 billion in annual revenue across 14 hospitals in three states: New Mexico, Oklahoma, and Texas.[33]

After closing the deal, Ventas separated Ardent's hospital operations from its real estate. Ventas took ownership of Ardent's real estate and sold a majority stake in its hospital operations to Equity Group Investments (EGI) for $475 million. Ventas retained a 9.9% interest in the hospital operations. Ardent's executive management team retained a significant equity stake. EGI is a private equity firm founded in 1968 by legendary investor Sam Zell. It is invested in energy, manufacturing, transportation, media, waste management, and real estate, as well as health care. It has spawned other companies such as Equity Residential, the largest apartment owner in the United States; Equity Office Properties Trust, the largest office owner in the country; and Equity Lifestyle Properties, an owner-operator of manufactured home and resort communities. EGI entered into a preagreed long-term triple-net lease with Ventas with an initial base rent of $105 million with annual escalators of 2.5%. A triple-net lease is a lease agreement on a property whereby the tenant pays all the expenses of the property, including real estate taxes, building insurance, utilities, and maintenance. With a triple-net lease, almost all responsibilities fall on the tenant. Lovelace Women's Hospital was now paying rent on property it once owned.

Ardent's "buy and build" business strategy included not only acquiring hospital systems and individual facilities but also engaging in joint ventures where Ardent would develop a partnership with nonprofit hospitals and academic medical centers. The joint venture would be structured to give Ardent a majority ownership interest (typically between 60% and 80%), the ability to charge a management fee in exchange for managing the day-to-day operations of the joint venture, and the right to receive a quarterly distribution of excess cash beyond required capital needs.

Under Ventas's and EGI's ownership, four acquisitions were completed—two in Texas, one in Oklahoma, and one in Kansas. Ardent describes these acquisitions:

In March 2017, we completed the acquisition of LHP, which owned and operated five hospitals and had partnerships with four significant not-for-profit systems and foundations in New Jersey, Texas, Florida and Idaho. The acquisition of LHP provided us immediate scale in growing markets and diversified our footprint into four new markets and three additional states. As a result of our acquisition of LHP, we currently own approximately 76% of a joint venture with Portneuf Health Trust (Portneuf Medical Center), 80% and 65% of joint ventures with Hackensack Meridian Health System (with respect to HackensackUMC Mountainside and HackensackUMC Pascack Valley facilities, respectively), 80% of a joint venture with Sacred Heart Health System / Ascension Health (Bay Medical Center Sacred Heart) and 80% of a joint venture with Seton Healthcare System / Ascension Health (Harker Heights).

Effective May 2017, we entered into a long-term lease agreement with the Mayes County Hospital Authority to assume operations and associated assets of AllianceHealth Pryor, a 52-bed hospital from Community Health Systems in Pryor, Oklahoma, for $0.9 million. Hillcrest subsequently renamed the hospital Hillcrest Hospital Pryor ("Pryor").

On November 1 2017, we completed the acquisition of St. Francis in Topeka, Kansas for $3.6 million, including acquired working capital, and entered into a related joint venture partnership with the University of Kansas Health System. The system, which includes a 378-bed hospital and 12 clinic locations, has been renamed the University of Kansas Health System St. Francis Campus (the "UKHS St. Francis Campus"). We own 75% of the joint venture and manage the operations of the health system.

Effective March 1, 2018, we completed the acquisition of nine hospitals, 52 clinics and other related ancillary operations of ETMC [East Texas Medical Center Regional Healthcare System] throughout Eastern Texas and entered into a joint venture agreement with UTHSCT [University of Texas Health Science Center at Tyler], an affiliate of the University of Texas System, which also has locations in Houston, San Antonio, Galveston and Dallas. We also entered into an agreement to manage the clinical operations of an additional hospital that was not acquired, the UT Health North Campus in Tyler, Texas ("UT Health North Campus Tyler"). The new 10-hospital regional health system was named UT Health East Texas ("UT Health East Texas"). We own 70% of the joint venture and manage the operations of the health system.[34]

Ardent's acquisitions under Ventas and EGI involved taking on additional debt. In March 2018, Ardent received a $300 million loan from Barclays Bank and Jefferies Finance. The company received another $1.63 million from OFS Capital, a business development company that primarily provides senior secured, floating-rate loans.[35]

On December 4, 2018, Ardent filed for an initial public offering (IPO) with the Securities and Exchange Commission and planned to list on the New York Stock Exchange (NYSE) under the symbol ARDT. An IPO allows a company to sell shares to and raise capital from public investors. A company filing for an IPO is required by the Securities and Exchange Commission to submit a prospectus, also known as an offer document. The prospectus helps investors get a picture of a company and make an informed decision to invest or not.

The purpose of the IPO Ardent filed on December 4, 2018, was not to exit the investment but to raise $100 million to pay down some of the debt it had accumulated over the years.[36]

The prospectus for the offering has several sections: use of proceeds (what the company intends to do with the capital); management (brief biographies of all the top management team members—chief executive officer, chief operating officer, chief financial officer, and the members of the board of directors); executive pay (base salaries and annual incentive compensation);

and summary of risk factors (the company's warnings to investors of internal and external factors that could cause the value of the stock to decrease).

In the section "Our Company," Ardent presents itself as "a leading provider of comprehensive, cost-effective quality health-care and related services in nine growing urban markets across Texas, New Mexico, Oklahoma, New Jersey, Idaho, Florida and Kansas." It further states, "As of September 30, 2018, we operated 31 acute care hospitals, including one managed hospital, two re-habilitation hospitals and two surgical hospitals, with a total of 4,718 licensed beds."[37]

Ardent's growth strategy is to expand services within its existing urban markets, improve operating margins of recent acquisi-tions, and pursue strategic acquisitions and joint venture oppor-tunities. It continues to invest in outpatient care facilities, urgent care facilities, and other ancillary services.

The weight of debt permeates the prospectus. The singular fo-cus on debt is not on its potential impact on hospital operations or the quality of health-care delivery but on its effect on the abil-ity to execute the business model: to consolidate, pay dividends, and divest assets.

In the section "Risks Related to Our Business and Industry," the prospectus reveals that Ardent has a significant amount of debt. As of September 30, 2018, Ardent's debt consisted of $475.0 million in outstanding senior notes, $822.9 million under a term loan B facility, $30.0 million under the ABL Facilities, and $7.3 million of other indebtedness. In addition, as of Sep-tember 30, 2018, it had the ability to draw an additional $171.5 mil-lion under the ABL Facilities.[38] Asset-based lending (ABL) is a loan where the assets of the borrowing company serve as collat-eral. The assets may be accounts receivable, inventory, or real estate. ABL loans are often used by companies with cash-flow problems.[39]

The prospectus acknowledges the significant threat Ardent's debt poses to the company, from the inability to fund basic operations to the potential for default. It states,

> Our substantial debt could have important consequences to us, including:
> - increasing our vulnerability to general economic and industry conditions;
> - requiring a substantial portion of our cash flow used in operations to be dedicated to the payment of principal and interest on our indebtedness, therefore reducing our liquidity and our ability to use our cash flow to fund our operations, capital expenditures and future business opportunities; . . .
> - limiting our ability to obtain additional financing for working capital, capital expenditures, debt service requirements, acquisitions and general corporate or other purposes;
> - limiting our ability to adjust to changing marketplace conditions and placing us at a competitive disadvantage compared to our competitors who may have less debt.[40]

In addition, there are conditions under which it could default on its debt.

Cross-default and cross-acceleration are provisions of a loan agreement designed to protect the lender. A default occurs when a borrower fails to make timely payments of principal or interest. A cross-default provision states that if a borrower defaults on one of its loans, it can be declared in default on another of its loans. For example, a cross-default clause in a loan agreement may say that if a person defaults on his car loan, he automatically defaults on his mortgage.

If a borrower defaults on a loan, the lender may accelerate repayment, making the loan due and payable before its scheduled maturation. A cross-acceleration provision effectively gives the lender of another loan the benefit of the acceleration provisions in the defaulted loan. If a borrower defaults on a car loan and the lender makes the loan due and payable, the lender of the mortgage, by cross-acceleration, can make the mortgage loan due and payable.

Ardent has multiple loans and lenders.

The prospectus sees this as an ominous possibility:

> Some of the instruments governing our existing indebtedness contain cross-default or cross-acceleration provisions that could result in our debt being declared immediately due and payable under a number of debt instruments, even if we default on only one debt instrument. In such event, it is unlikely that we would be able to satisfy our obligations under all of such accelerated indebtedness simultaneously.
>
> There are no assurances that we will maintain a level of liquidity sufficient to permit us to pay the principal, premium and interest on our indebtedness or to grow our business and use our capital effectively.
>
> As of September 30, 2018, we had $852.9 million, or approximately 63.9%, of our outstanding total debt at variable interest rates. If interest rates increase, our debt service obligations on our variable rate indebtedness will increase even though the amount borrowed remains the same, and therefore net income and associated cash flows, including cash available for servicing our indebtedness, will correspondingly decrease. Effective August 31, 2018, we have executed interest rate swaps with Barclays Bank PLC and Bank of America, N.A., as counterparties, with notional amounts totaling $558.0 million, expiring August 31, 2023. We have entered into these agreements to manage our exposure to fluctuations in interest rates.[41]

The prospectus states that the agreements that govern its existing indebtedness—the cross-default and cross-acceleration provisions and the variable rates—could impose significant operating and financial restrictions:

These restrictions will limit our ability and the ability of our subsidiaries to, among other things:

. . .

- pay dividends and make other distributions on, or redeem or repurchase, capital stock;
- make certain investments; . . .
- enter into transactions with affiliates;
- merge or consolidate;
- enter into agreements that restrict the ability of our subsidiaries to make dividends or other payments to us; . . .
- transfer or sell assets.

. . . As a result of these restrictions, we will be limited as to how we conduct our business and we may be unable to raise additional debt or equity financing to compete effectively or to take advantage of new business opportunities.[42]

On June 28, 2018, while the IPO was in process, Ardent refinanced its existing debt in an attempt to improve its financial picture. The refinancing transactions included $990 million in new senior secured credit facilities. In addition, Ardent subsidiary AHP Health Partners would issue up to $535 million of senior unsecured notes, which would be due in 2026.[43] An unsecured note is a loan that is not secured by the issuer's assets. Because they are not backed by collateral and are riskier prospects for an investor, the interest rates offered are higher than for secured debt. The notes and the guarantees were offered in a private offering.[44] Net proceeds from the transactions would be used to refinance or extinguish Ardent's existing credit facilities and provide working capital for general corporate purposes.

In connection with the refinancing transactions, Ardent incurred a loss on debt extinguishment of $47.7 million. "A loss on extinguishment of debt occurs when there is a difference between the repurchase price and the carrying amount of debt at the time of extinguishment."[45] The repurchase price is the amount the debt holder pays to extinguish the debt. The carrying amount of debt is the amount that would have been payable at the maturity date. A loss on the extinguishment of a debt occurs when the repurchase price to eradicate the debt is greater than the amount of the debt at maturity. Ardent paid $47.7 million to pay off the debt.[46]

An analysis of the prospectus and the IPO, "Ardent Health IPO Was Organized to Get Out of Debt," was published by Bilbao Asset Management on December 11, 2018. It contained several warnings for prospective investors.

According to the analysis, investors should be concerned about Ardent's massive amount of debt and liability:

> As of September 30, 2018, the long-term debt obligations including interest were more than $2 billion. Ardent Health reported this amount of debt assuming an interest rate of 7.73%. The list of contractual obligations shows that Ardent will need to pay $323 million in less than a year, $635 million in one to three years. Taking into account the total amount of cash in hand as of today, Ardent Health will have troubles to pay these sums. It is clear that further financing is needed to pay these debts.[47]

Another concern was Ardent's intention to be a controlled company with a nonindependent board of directors. The corporate governance rules of the NYSE require that a company's board of directors consist of a majority of independent directors and that the compensation committee and the nominating and corporate governance committees be composed entirely of independent directors. Under NYSE rules, however, a company of which more than 50% of the voting power for the election of directors is held by an individual, a group, or another company is a "controlled company" and may elect not to comply with certain corporate governance requirements. EGI is, and would continue to be, the controlling stockholder of Ardent. Because Ardent's controlling stockholder would continue to control a majority of the combined voting power of its common stock after completion of this offering, Ardent stated it would be a controlled company. This would exempt it from having to comply with NYSE corporate governance rules. The prospectus notes,

> Because our controlling stockholder will continue to control a majority of the combined voting power of our common stock after completion of this offering, we will be a "controlled company" within the meaning of the corporate governance standards of the NYSE. Under these rules, a company of which more than 50% of the voting power for the election of directors is held by an individual, group or another company is a "controlled company" and may elect not to comply with certain corporate governance requirements, including the requirements that, within one year of the date of the listing of our common stock:
> - we have a Board that is composed of a majority of independent directors, as defined under the listing rules of the NYSE;
> - we have a compensation committee that is composed entirely of independent directors; and
> - we have a nominating and corporate governance committee that is composed entirely of independent directors.
>
> For at least a period of time following this offering, we intend to utilize these exemptions. As a result, we will not have a majority of independent directors and our nominating and corporate governance committee and compensation committee will not consist entirely of independent directors.[48]

The Bilbao analysis explains that minority shareholders should understand that Ardent's status as a controlled company with a nonindependent board of directors meant the board could make decisions to benefit the largest shareholders, contrary to the interest of minority shareholders. In the prospectus, Ardent concedes as much, stating that its status as a controlled company could make its common stock less attractive to some investors. The prospectus warns investors that they would not have the same protections afforded to stockholders of companies that are subject to all of the corporate governance requirements of the NYSE and have independent directors. The prospectus speaks directly to investors:

> The interests of EGI and Ventas, our two largest stockholders, may conflict with yours. . . . Accordingly, EGI has the ability to influence significantly our policies and operations, and its interests may not in all cases be aligned with your interests. For example, EGI may have an interest in pursuing acquisitions, divestitures, financings or other transactions that, in their judgment, could enhance their equity investment, even though such transactions might involve risks to you as a stockholder.[49]

"Liquidity" refers to the level of cash on hand or a company's ability to convert assets to cash to pay its short-term obligations or liabilities. Strong liquidity means there's enough cash to pay off any debts that may arise. The Bilbao analysis found that Ardent's "financial shape does not seem quite beneficial. With $60 million in cash and accounts receivable of $534 million, Ardent Health may find liquidity issues in the future, which the market should not appreciate."[50]

The Bilbao analysis concludes that given its contractual obligations and massive debt; that the use of the proceeds from the IPO will be used to repay debt; and that, as Ardent is a controlled company, the board of directors could make decisions that benefit the largest shareholders and are damaging to the interests of minority investors, "Ardent Health does not seem appealing."[51]

Debt may be the lifeblood of private equity, but it can be crippling to the ambitions of the private equity firm. IASIS Healthcare was created as a health-care platform company in 1999 by private equity firm JLL Partners. The hospital system grew by adding on hospitals in geographically dispersed health markets in Arizona, Colorado, Louisiana, Texas, and Utah. In 2004, the private equity firm Texas Pacific Group acquired a majority stake in IASIS by a $1.5 billion leveraged buyout. On February 4, 2015, IASIS filed for an IPO with the Securities and Exchange Commission. The company said it would use cash from the IPO to pay off debts and regain its footing as a for-profit company. The IPO proved not to be attractive to public market investors. On December 30, 2016, the last business day of the year, IASIS announced the cancellation of the IPO. The failure of the IPO was due to IASIS's extensive junk bond debt. In 2011 IASIS had sold more than $450 million in junk bonds that increased its debt burden from 4.9 to 6.5 times earnings. Over $230 million of the junk bond sale was a dividend recapitalization payout to IASIS's private equity owners.[52]

On January 8, 2020, Ardent withdrew its IPO. Ardent did not disclose a reason for the withdrawal.

5

Moral Agency

In his book *Beyond Caring: Hospitals, Nurses, and the Social Organization of Ethics*, sociologist Daniel Chambliss writes, "The discipline of bioethics, expanded from medical ethics, has bypassed nursing."[1] He cites Paul Ramsey's classic book *The Patient as Person: Explorations in Medical Ethics*, which has no mention of nursing in its index. He also cites a major handbook, *Clinical Ethics*, which doesn't have an index but does have a "locator" where there are listings for "patient-physician relationship" and "physician responsibility" but nothing for nursing. He concludes that this should not be considered unreasonable because medical ethics are geared primarily to physicians. Chambliss argues that nursing, although it carries out ethical decisions, has no place in the discussion. Ethics are for powerful people who make decisions, not the powerless who carry them out. Nurses are subordinated in hospitals in several ways: subject to institutional policies, to directives by supervisors and administrators, to the orders of physicians. They are required to work within the doctor's vision of the patient's diagnosis, treatment, and expectations. Nurses are often compelled to carry out orders with which they disagree, treatments they believe to be unnecessary, even cruel. "Nursing ethics, then, is the ethics of powerless people; the ethics of witnesses, not decision makers; the ethics of implementers, not choosers; the ethics of those whose work goes unnoticed."[2]

In 1980, brothers Stuart E. Dreyfus, an applied mathematician, and Hubert L. Dreyfus, a philosopher, submitted an 18-page research report to the United States Air Force Office of Scientific Research at the University of California, Berkeley. Now known as the Dreyfus model of skill acquisition, it was based on the study of chess masters, air force pilots, and army tank drivers and commanders. The Dreyfus brothers believed students learned through experience and passed through five distinct stages: novice, advanced beginner, competent, proficient, and expert.[3]

In 1984, the nurse theorist Patricia Benner published *From Novice to Expert: Excellence and Power in Clinical Nursing Practice*.[4] The book was based on a study using the Dreyfus model. The study was conducted between 1978 and 1981 and spanned the spectrum of nursing. It was based on interviews with and participant observation of 11 newly graduated nurses and their preceptors, 51 experienced nurse clinicians, and 5 senior nursing students in six hospitals: two private community hospitals, two teaching hospitals, one university medical center, and one inner-city general hospital. Benner's method was largely to work with nurses in small groups where they would give narrative accounts of clinical situations and describe how they provided patient care, made clinical decisions, and managed patients, families, colleagues, and physicians. Hubert and Stuart Dreyfus served as consultants in the study.

Theories of nursing range from the abstract, such as Margaret Newman's theory of health as expanding consciousness or Rosemarie Parse's theory of human becoming, to the esoteric. Martha Rogers's theory, the science of unitary human beings, states that human beings are irreducible, indivisible energy fields without spatial or temporal attributes. They are open for exchange and extend to infinity. There are eight concepts in Rogers's theory: energy field, openness, pattern, pandimensionality, hemodynamic principles, resonance, helicy, and integrality.[5]

Benner's nursing theory is about practice.

One of the central tenets of Benner's *From Novice to Expert* is that "we cannot get beyond experience," be responsible for what has not yet been encountered in practice.[6] Experience is more than the passage of time, more than encountering medical conditions and situations. Experience is when the situation you encounter is different from what theory predicted or led you to expect. Only when the situation changes, elaborates, or disconfirms preconceived notions does experience happen. Experience is the refinement of theory by the real.

Experience leads to expertise. The experience of seeing many patients in a similar situation creates narrative memories. It leads to an immediate intuitive grasp of the clinical situation. The nurse sees what needs to be done without having to go through an analytical process. Expert nurses read the patient and respond instantaneously. Clinical grasp and clinical response are inextricably linked. Benner describes expert nursing as seamless performance, fluid, nonreflective.

Expert nurses have what Benner calls the skill of involvement. The nurse-patient relationship is a changing pattern of intimacy and distance in some of the most dramatic, poignant, and painful moments of life. In the narratives in Benner's study, nurses spoke about the right kind of relationship with patients and families, how close to be. Getting it right means having the right distance, understanding their needs and wishes. Expert nurses have an increased level of emotional involvement and moral connection with patients and families. They monitor not only the patient's response to illness and treatment but also the patient's suffering, resourcefulness, and possibilities. They understand the expectations of families, recognize signs of trust, hostility, and anger. They learn how to share information with families that conveys the gravity of the situation yet reserves their right to hope and have faith that everything that should be done is being done.

Involvement leads to moral agency. Expert nurses have a sense of responsibility and self-efficacy. They see themselves as participating members of the health-care team. The expert nurse develops a moral voice and an advocacy for and solidarity with patients and families. Hubert and Stuart Dreyfus saw the expert nurse as an independent ethical actor having a high level of clinical autonomy. Subordination is only one way of looking at nursing. In her book *Devices and Desires: Gender, Technology, and American Nursing*, Margarete Sandelowski describes the role nurses have played in the implementation of medical technology: "Nurses were indispensable to the early-twentieth-century scientific and technological transformation of health care and medicine in the United States."[7] She sees nurses as the infrastructure of medical technology because of how they have positioned themselves between patient and machine. She describes this as the "in-betweenness" of nurses. She refers to them as "quintessential boundary workers, regularly crossing the terrain between the patient and physician, disease and illness, and medical world and everyday practices."[8] In-betweenness opens up spaces and possibilities for nursing practice.

The appropriate use of technological interventions was a theme in many of the expert narratives in Benner's study. They described the experience of patients whose dying and suffering were prolonged by therapeutic relentlessness. They expressed a recognition of the limits of medical heroism, of the possibilities for harm in overzealous treatment. They saw themselves as a buffer against medical zeal, against the view identified by Ira Byock, who wrote, "A strong presumption throughout my medical education was that

all seriously ill people required vigorous life-prolonging treatment, including those who were expected to die, even patients
with advanced chronic illness. It even extended to patients who
saw death as a relief from the suffering caused by their illness."[9]

Usually nurses are aligned with the medical plan. They share
the physician's vision of the patient. Medicine is the wind in their
sails. But sometimes they don't share that vision. They tack and
sail against the wind. From their experience, from their emotional
and clinical relationship with the patient, expert nurses are able
to see the likely future. They can recognize the distinction between reasonable heroic efforts and unreasonable, futile care
that prolongs suffering and dying. They know the good for the
patient even if it's death.

Expert nurses are able to achieve their ends despite structural
limitations that constrict their practice. Nurses can't order MRIs
or digoxin or a swallow study, but they can influence the clinical
situation. Benner describes moral agency as working with and
through others.[10] In their essay "Nurses Must Be Clever to Care,"
Sanchia Aranda and Rosie Brown refer to the complex work of
nurses, which takes place in private spaces with the patient and
the family and which involves skills that are often hidden from
view. The intimacy and trust between the expert nurse and the
family, the moral bond, creates possibilities—what can be thought
about and talked about. In quiet places not seen, the nurse works
with and through families to bring about the good, what is best
for the patient.[11] "When we get sick," Suzanne Gordon writes, "we
are supposed to become characters in a heroic medical narrative
that conceals the remorselessness of pathology, the intractable
fact of human vulnerability, and the inevitable inadequacies of
medicine."[12] The expert nurse can change that narrative. One day
a patient told me that the hospitalist said that the ICU nurses think
they're doctors but they're not. But I read their notes, look at the
imaging they look at, the labs. Hear what they say to the family.

Medicine veils death. It deconstructs it from an unthinkable possibility into a series of small, manageable, biomedical problems: heart rate, blood pressure, urine output that the physician can "fix." The nurse can unveil it. Before you die, you're dying. In-betweenness. You leave the land of medicine and cross the terrain to the land of the family. Moral agency is an ethic of protection. It involves advocacy, defense, rescue.

6

Do No Harm

There is a harm in health care we should not do, of which Hippocrates wrote in *Of the Epidemics*, "First, do no harm" (Primum non nocere), and Florence Nightingale, in *Notes on Hospitals*, wrote, "The very first requirement in a hospital is that it should do the sick no harm."[1] A 2016 study by Johns Hopkins "claims more than 250,000 people in the U.S. die every year from medical errors. Medical errors are the third-leading cause of death after heart disease and cancer."[2]

Early American hospitals were for the "worthy poor," for people who had no family or were away from home. They were more charitable than medical institutions. Physicians had little impact on the daily life of the hospital. There was little in the way of therapeutics. Therapy was "diet, rest, and the healing power of nature."[3] Patients were there for months, even years. A mid-nineteenth-century hospital was more like a well-run boarding house.

Then came the discovery of bacteria, antibiotics, sterilization, anesthesia. Technology. In 1850 the ophthalmoscope. In 1857 the laryngoscope. In 1895 the X-ray. The ability to diagnose. The hospital was medicalized. It became a place for treatment. It was possible to be cured. And harmed.

The rubric is "patient safety event," which is an event that could have resulted or did result in harm to a patient. It has its own lexicon.

> An error is defined as the failure of a planned action to be completed as intended (i.e., error of execution) or the use of a wrong plan to achieve an aim (i.e., error of planning). An adverse event is an injury caused by medical management rather than the underlying condition of the patient. An adverse event attributable to error is a "preventable adverse event." Negligent adverse events represent a subset of preventable adverse events that satisfy legal criteria used in determining negligence (i.e., whether the care provided failed to meet the standard of care reasonably expected of an average physician qualified to take care of the patient in question).[4]

Patient safety events also include no-harm events, near misses, and hazardous conditions.

It became a question of not just whether a hospital provides good medical care, but whether it is safe. The Joint Commission on Accreditation of Hospitals was founded in 1951 as a private organization that evaluated and accredited hospitals and other health-care organizations. It began with the efforts of pioneering Boston surgeon Ernest Amory Codman, who is the "acknowledged founder of what today is known as outcomes management in patient care."[5]

The commission "was created by merging the American College of Surgeons Hospital Standardization Program with similar programs run by the American College of Physicians, the American Hospital Association, the American Medical Association, and the Canadian Medical Association."[6]

It wasn't until 1965, when the federal government decided that a hospital that was accredited by the Joint Commission met the

Medicare Conditions of Participation for the receipt of Medicaid and Medicare reimbursements, that accreditation had any official impact. In 1987 it was renamed the Joint Commission on Accreditation of Healthcare Organizations. In 2007, it simplified its name to the Joint Commission. Its slogan was, "Helping health care organizations help patients." Its goal is to support quality improvement and patient safety in health-care organizations.[7] Every year the commission issues National Patient Safety Goals that highlight problematic areas and provide evidence-based solutions.

In 1996, the Joint Commission announced the Sentinel Event Policy.[8] It defined a sentinel event as an unexpected occurrence that resulted in death or serious physical or psychological injury. Examples of sentinel events are wrong-site, wrong-procedure, wrong-patient surgery; patient death or injury in restraints; transfusion error; operative or postoperative complication; unexpected death of a full-term infant; and radiation therapy to the wrong body region or 25% above the planned dose. Such events are called "sentinel" because they signal the need for immediate investigation. Hospitals are encouraged, but not required, to report sentinel events to the Joint Commission. The commission offers support and expertise during the review of the sentinel event and the opportunity to collaborate with a patient safety expert. The Joint Commission does mandate performance of a root cause analysis within 45 calendar days of a sentinel event. "Failure to perform an RCA within 45 days of a sentinel event may result in the healthcare institution being placed on an accreditation watch, which is public information."[9]

Then there are "never events."[10] The National Quality Forum (NQF), established in 1999, is a nonprofit membership organization with the goal of promoting patient safety and health-care quality through performance measurement and public reporting. The NQF's membership includes over 400 organizations representing consumers, health plans, medical professionals, employers, public health agencies, and medical device companies. The NQF uses consensus-based national standards to measure whether health-care performance is safe, timely, beneficial, patient centered, equitable, and efficient. In 2002, the NQF published *Serious Reportable Events in Healthcare: A Consensus Report*. It was a list of 28 medical events that are so egregious and preventable that they should never happen to a patient. They later became known as "never events." The list includes such events as patient death or serious injury from contaminated drugs, patient suicide, preventable postoperative death, and patient death or serious disability associated with a fall. The NQF contends that the risk of occurrence of a never event is significantly influenced by the policies and procedures of the health-care organization. According to Debra L. Ness, president of the National Partnership for Women and Families, "Never events are a symptom of a health care system that is broken and unresponsive."[11] The NQF's never events are also considered sentinel events by the Joint Commission. In August 2007, the Centers for Medicare and Medicaid Services announced that Medicare would no longer pay for additional costs associated with never events.

On November 29, 1999, the Institute of Medicine released a report titled *To Err Is Human: Building a Safer Health System*.[12] The report stated that medical errors in American hospitals cause as many as 98,000 deaths every year. The message of *To Err Is Human* was that caring, responsible, competent health-care professionals could make honest mistakes. To err is human. The problem was not that there were bad people in health care, but that good people were working in bad systems that needed to be made safer. Its calls for hospital reform received national media attention and led to congressional hearings. The report called for a 50% reduction in medical errors over five years. It concluded with four recommendations, one of which urged health-care organizations to build a culture of safety and to adopt safety principles known in other industries.

The concept of safety culture originated outside health care, in studies of high-reliability organizations (HROs). HROs are organizations that consistently minimize adverse events despite carrying out intrinsically complex and hazardous work. They maintain a commitment to safety at all levels, from frontline providers to managers and executives.[13] Nuclear power operations, wildland firefighting, and air traffic control are examples. HRO research includes studies of disasters: Three Mile Island, the *Challenger* explosion, the Black Hawk friendly fire incident in Iraq. In hospitals, the operating room, the emergency department, and the ICU are HROs.

HROs have five characteristics:

(1) sensitivity to operations (*ie*, heightened awareness of the state of relevant systems and processes); (2) reluctance to simplify (*ie*, the acceptance that work is complex, with the potential to fail in new and unexpected ways); (3) preoccupation with failure (*ie*, to view near misses as opportunities to improve, rather than proof of success); (4) deference to expertise (*ie*, to value insights from staff with the most pertinent safety knowledge over those with greater seniority); (5) and practicing resilience (*ie*, to prioritize emergency training for many unlikely, but possible, system failures).[14]

In his 1997 book, *Managing the Risks of Organizational Accidents*, James Reason postulated the idea of just culture as one of the components of a safety culture.[15] "Just culture originated in the 1980s in the aviation industry where safety errors can have catastrophic results."[16]

To reduce the risk of aircraft accidents, the industry thoroughly reviewed its technology, training, and aviation culture. It found that the conditions for accidents were often well known by people in the workplace, but those individuals were afraid to speak up for fear of retaliation or punishment. Critical information about unsafe conditions was driven underground. The review led to a cultural shift that focused on systems rather than blame, moving from asking, "Who made the mistake?" to asking, "What went wrong?" Just culture in the aviation industry encourages and rewards individuals for bringing forward safety concerns.

In a blame culture, errors are the fault of an individual who can be fired or punished for the error. In a blame-free culture, all errors are considered to have their roots in the system. "A just culture is the opposite of a blame culture, but it is not the same as a no-blame culture."[17] It is a culture of accountability. Although just culture recognizes the virtue of "no blame," certain errors are the result of incompetency, carelessness, or recklessness and merit blame and disciplinary action. A just culture focuses on identifying and addressing systems issues that lead individuals to engage in unsafe behaviors, while maintaining individual accountability by establishing zero tolerance for reckless behavior.[18] A just culture distinguishes between human error, at-risk behavior, and reckless behavior. Giving the wrong amount of morphine is human error. Not taking a time-out before surgery, even if the patient is unharmed, is reckless behavior.

On March 1, 2017, the Joint Commission issued "Sentinel Event Alert 57: The Essential Role of Leadership in Developing a Safety Culture."[19] The Joint Commission has a Sentinel Event Database that collects reports from organizations that have experienced a sentinel event. The data is analyzed to identify the root causes of the events. The database revealed a correlation between the failure of leadership to create an effective safety culture and adverse events ranging from wrong-site surgery to delays in treatment. The Joint Commission saw leadership as integral to and responsible for the development of a safety culture. Leaders guide the transition from a culture of blame, intimidation, and fear of retaliation to an organization with open communication, mutual trust, and a shared perception of the importance of safety.

7

Behind the Curtain

I usually get to the unit a little before seven. I say hi to Jill, the night secretary. She's in nursing school at the University of New Mexico. She's always happy to see me because it means she can go home. I put the lights on in the nurses' station. Say, "Sun's up." Look at the board to see how many patients, what status they are. There's one computer I like because it raises up high, so I find it and put my clipboard on it. Gavin usually comes in right after. He's our charge nurse. The first thing he does is empty the trash in the nurses' station because it's always overflowing. I think this habit comes from doing chores. He lives on a farm in the East Mountains. Kristen comes in after Gavin. She came to the ICU from Med-Surg two years ago. In nursing, there's days, nights, the front of the week, the back of the week. Gavin, Kristen, and I work days, the front of the week. We're a team. There's a large whiteboard on the back wall. It has squares separated with black tape. Different squares have the patient's initials, service, diagnosis, level of care (ICU or Intermediate Care), who the nurse is, code status, then things like if they're on a ventilator, if they're on isolation. The night charge and Gavin stand by the board and the charge gives

Gavin report patient by patient. Gavin writes the assignments on the board with a black Sharpie, the day nurse's name above the night nurse's. Sometimes he'll check with me or Kristen about the assignments and ask, "You good?" Starting a shift is like getting on a moving train. Shift change is like the train is going through a small town so it's moving slowly. It'll pick up speed when it gets through the town. You get report from the night nurse. You step onto the train. I do the same thing every day. I open the patient's chart, look at the past medical history, what they presented with, the admitting diagnosis, the physician progress notes, the plan, any events, the diagnostic tests (CT, X-ray, labs). If the tests are abnormal, I look at previous labs because we treat trends, not numbers. I try to get a picture and a sense of which way things are going. Then I go into the room to the side of the bed and introduce myself. Now the train's picking up speed. It's a 12-hour trip. There won't be any stops. From the train, the outside world is a blur. Your world is the train. Your patients. Families. Tasks. Procedures.

I never thought much about who owned the hospital where I worked, how it was run, whether there was a president or a board of directors. I know the University of New Mexico Hospital (UNM) and Presbyterian are local. I know UNM used to be called the Bernalillo County Indian Hospital because it was built on land donated by the Bureau of Indian Affairs on the condition that the hospital maintain at least 100 beds for Native American patients. Presbyterian was originally a sanatorium. It was founded by Rev. Hugh A. Cooper, a Presbyterian pastor. The Presbyterian administration building is named after him. It's nicknamed the "Coop." Presbyterian is a statewide system with hospitals in Clovis, Espanola, Rio Rancho, Ruidoso, Socorro, and Tucumcari and two in Albuquerque. Lovelace isn't local. I know it's owned by a company named Ardent Health Services based in Nashville, Tennessee. I didn't know where the name Lovelace came from.

Private equity companies are behind a curtain. When they buy a company, they don't have to notify anybody: employees, unions, vendors. On April 6, 2015, when the private equity company Ventas agreed to buy Ardent Health Services, we didn't know about it.

It was Levophed that gave me the first glimpse behind the curtain.

The ICU is different from other nursing units. The patients are sicker. There are skills ICU nurses have that other nurses don't. You need to have advanced cardiac life support certification. You need to know the algorithms for life-threatening arrhythmias and cardiac arrest that you use in codes. You need to know how to manage a ventilator, interpret an arterial blood gas analysis. You need to know drugs that infuse into the body. We call them drips. We can raise your blood pressure with Levophed. Lower it with Nipride. We can make the heart contract harder with dobutamine. Make it slower with Cardizem. We can sedate you with Ativan. Paralyze you with Nimbex. Drips can save your life, but they can also harm you. You can get cyanide toxicity from Nipride. Dopamine can make your heart race. Drips are almost the heart and soul of ICU nursing. Nurses have to know them inside out. If a patient is on a drip, they can't be on the floor. They have to be in the ICU.

R. Adams Cowley, a pioneer in open-heart surgery, is considered the father of trauma medicine. In 1958, he founded the R. Adams Cowley Shock Trauma Center, referred to simply as Shock Trauma, at the University of Maryland Medical Center. It had a small staff. Two, later four, beds. It was known as the "death lab" until patients given up for dead began to survive. It was the first facility in the world to treat shock.[1]

Shock is when blood pressure is too low and organs and tissues aren't receiving an adequate flow of oxygenated blood. Cowley described shock as a "momentary pause in the act of death."[2] Shock is one of the leading causes of death in the ICU. There are different kinds. In cardiogenic shock, the heart can't pump enough blood to the body. Bacteria in the blood—bacteremia—causes septic shock. Severe blood loss leads to hemorrhagic shock.

The first-line drug in the ICU for the treatment of shock is Levophed. Levophed is a vasopressor. Vasopressors constrict blood vessels. This causes resistance to blood flow from the heart, which in turn causes an increase in blood pressure and increased perfusion to vital organs: the heart, brain, lungs. Of all the medications we infuse in the ICU, Levophed is the most powerful. A receptor is a molecule to which a drug binds that initiates a physiological response. Beta 1 receptors stimulate the heart. Beta 2 the lungs. Alpha 1 receptors cause vasoconstriction of arteries and veins. Levophed is almost pure alpha. The vasoconstriction it induces is so extreme it can cause ischemia of the fingers and toes. They can become necrotic, turn black. We mark the borders every day to see if the necrosis is advancing, so each toe has a unique squiggly tattoo. Sometimes they need to be amputated. We call the drug "leave 'em dead Levophed."

Drugs are infused in different ways. Dopamine is weight based, micrograms per kilogram per minute (mcg/kg/min). Vecuronium is milligrams per hour. Insulin is units per hour. Levophed is micrograms per minute (mcg/min). Nurses know the doses by heart. We have a pharmacist in the unit. One day he told us the dosing of Levophed had been changed to mcg/kg/min. Weight based. He said it came from administration and would be standardized for all Ardent hospitals.

Every profession has its own jargon. I read a story about a cardiologist who was piloting a plane from Phoenix to San Diego. He was in distress. He was in touch with the air traffic controller, who could see he was flying too low and kept telling him he needed to ascend. The air traffic controller warned he was still losing altitude and told him, "I need you to fly." He plowed into a San Diego neighborhood, killing a UPS driver and two elderly people in their home. Afterward, the controller said he thought the pilot was struggling with a distraction but did not communicate it to air traffic control. The controller said, "The first thing you do when you're in trouble is call, climb and confess—and he did not do any of the three."[3] Call, climb, confess. Jargon isn't just language, it's liturgy. It has a purpose. Brevity. Understanding. Guidance. We have our own jargon. Patients can "buck the vent," they "poop out on CPAP," they "flip" into atrial fibrillation, they "eat up" their platelets. They get "bronched," "Swanned," "tapped." In the crisis-laden atmosphere of the ICU, someone will ask, "What's the levo at?" And someone will respond, "Twelve." Everyone knows what that means. The max dose is 20, so you know you have some room. That understanding is lost when the response is, "They're on point two." The difference cannot be underestimated.

Someone changed the liturgy.

Levophed comes in a small plastic bag the size of a wallet. You know the numbers like you know your social security number. Four milligrams of Levophed in 250 ccs of normal saline is 0.016 milligrams per cc. To convert it to micrograms, you multiply by 1,000 and you get 16 micrograms per cc. Divided by 60 because it's given in minutes gives you a calculation factor of 0.266, which makes 1 mcg/min 3.75 ccs an hour, so you know that 10 mcg/min is 37 ccs an hour and 20 mcg/min is 74 ccs an hour. You can walk into the room, eyeball the pump, and know how much is infusing. Micrograms per minute is the universal language of Levophed. There were mistakes right away.

We admitted a patient from the emergency room in septic shock on a Levophed drip. During the handoff, the ER nurse said the patient was on 0.1 mcg/kg/min. When we looked at how the pump was programmed, we discovered it was running at 0.01 and her systolic pressure was a dangerously low 78. Three days later a patient came to us from the emergency room on a weight-based Levophed drip that converted to 38 mcg/min, far in excess of the maximum dose of 20 mcg/min, and the systolic pressure was within a normal range of 128.

The research doesn't support weight-based dosing of Levophed. A National Institutes of Health study concluded that not only was there no advantage in such dosing in the critically ill patient, there were potential disadvantages.[4] Weight-based dosing increases the complexity of care and can lead to medication errors, especially if not accurate. We use initial weight to titrate drips. Initial weight is what you weigh when you're admitted to the hospital, your normal weight before you start getting IV fluids. One of the first things you do to patients admitted to the hospital is weigh them and record it in the electronic medical record. Body weight has implications for how medications are metabolized, utilized, and stored. The average adult body is 60% water. Normally, most of it is stored in three spaces: the intracellular space, the intravascular space, and a small amount in the interstitial space, with the intracellular space holding about two-thirds of total body water. Patients who have received a lot of fluid can become fluid overloaded. When there's too much fluid, it moves from the blood into the interstitial space, the nonfunctional area between cells in organs and tissues that usually holds minimal fluid. It's called third-spacing. It's a false weight, not a true weight.

The complexity of care is that you don't always know the patient's weight. You have to find it in the electronic medical record. It's not always recorded. Then you have to weigh them, but it's not the initial weight. There are delays in weight-based protocols that do not exist for non-weight-based. The logistical necessity of finding the weight and then programming it into the infusion pump invites error and delay. It takes time. Time is everything in critical care. If you have a stroke, the time from arriving in the ER to getting tPA (tissue plasminogen activator) to break up the clot is called door-to-needle. If you have a heart attack, the time to getting a stent is door-to-balloon. Door-to-needle time is 30 minutes. Door-to-balloon is 90 minutes. If your stroke is more than 12 hours old, you can't get tPA. Too much time has gone by. With weight-based programming, nurses have to stop and think. In the ICU, a patient can die in a minute. A patient can die in the minute the nurse has to stop and think.

Shared governance in nursing was first popularized in 1984 with the publication of *Shared Governance for Nursing: A Creative Approach to Professional Accountability*.[5] Shared decision-making between bedside nurses and nurse administrators on issues such as clinical protocols, new equipment, and staffing was thought to promote a more positive culture, job satisfaction, and nurse retention. One of the authors, Tim Porter-O'Grady, defined it as a structural model through which nurses can manage their practice with a high level of professional autonomy. He later described it more succinctly as "control over practice."[6] Shared governance puts the responsibility, authority, and accountability for decisions about nursing practice into the hands of the nurses who will operationalize the decision. Decision-making is made by those at the point of care. Only 10% of unit-level decisions should be made by management. Both Med-Surg and the ICU at Lovelace Women's Hospital had shared governance. We met once a month. We wrote a mission statement. We had a leader, a facilitator, and a scribe. We read articles on how shared governance worked in other hospitals. We were working on changing the insulin protocol for diabetic ketoacidosis. It was hard. People had to come in on their days off. Do research on their own. Kids coming home from school. We were a start-up.

Before changing a policy or process, high reliability organizations look for possible adverse consequences. The method is called failure modes and effects analysis. Failure mode involves identifying possible problems that could occur with the change; effects analysis examines the consequences

This change in dosing came out of the blue.

The nursing office is on the first floor, just before the cafeteria. The door is locked. You have to swipe your badge to get in. On your left is a row of small rooms. A secretary's office, an office for the house supervisors, one for the unit educators. On the right is a big space with a round table where all the managers and the house supervisors "huddle" every change of shift. The office of the chief nursing officer (CNO) is in the very back. She's only been CNO a few years. She had been the assistant to the one who was fired. We're about the same age. She had been an oncology nurse. It's a small hospital, so I see her often in the cafeteria. Sometimes she does executive rounds. I told her about the Levophed errors in the ER admissions, that it was unsafe, that there was potential for patient harm. Evidence-based research didn't support it. She listened. I asked her who ordered the dosing change, what was used as evidence, and said that it should have gone through shared governance. "It was corporate," she said.

The New American Workplace was published by Eileen Appelbaum and Rosemary Batt in 1994. It was based on research on the relationship between a company's management and workers. They recognized a historical change in that relationship. The belief that investing in workers increased productivity and profit began to fray as companies began to outsource, "subcontracting parts of their businesses—accounting departments, cafeterias, janitorial services—rather than employing those workers directly."[7] Appelbaum and Batt found that the impetus for these practices was coming from Wall Street shareholders. "People had a very old view of what the corporation was, as a kind of stand-alone, publicly traded entity, free to make decisions on its own," Batt said. "We understood globalization, deregulation, and labor markets, but we didn't understand capital markets. There was this big hole in the academic research."[8] Capital markets are where people or companies with capital to lend or invest supply it to businesses that need it. Private equity is a capital market.

Appelbaum and Batt decided to focus their research on private equity funds. "They endeavored to write a book about private equity aimed at people who dealt with labor issues, including union leaders, who often didn't realize that, when they were negotiating with corporations over contracts and working conditions, the managers of private-equity firms were actually pulling the strings."[9]

I left the CNO's office thinking, *Someone else is pulling the strings.*

In July 2015, I didn't know what Ventas was. What private equity is. But I remember it as a time when things changed. The CNO had been fired. The ICU manager quit. We would have four managers over the next five years. The hospital announced a policy of whiteboards in patient rooms. The Affordable Care Act linked patient satisfaction to Medicare reimbursement. Whiteboards were said to improve patients' awareness of their care team and improve overall satisfaction. At the beginning of your shift, you would write a bunch of stuff on the whiteboard: your name, the name of the physician, the patient's diet, the patient's main concern, the goal for the day, the schedule of pain medication, when it was administered, when the next dose was due. If you didn't keep your whiteboard current, you were written up. Petty things. The hospital installed security cameras in the supply room we shared with Med-Surg as if we were stealing bandages and toothpaste. Vendors were changed for supplies. Urinals went from the translucent plastic to a nonabsorbent cardboard-type material so you couldn't see the color or turbidity of the urine. The new IV-start kits were flimsy and there was no flash of blood so you couldn't tell if you were in the vein. Long-tenured, senior nurses were told their salary was "maxed" and they would no longer receive annual raises. We had a four-person maintenance staff. I called them the Beatles. Two were fired. They had worked at Women's for years. People began to leave. I would go to Med-Surg and ask where so-and-so was and they would say, "Oh, she went to UNM," or "She's working at the VA."

Rather than hire new staff, they would float us from the ICU to Med-Surg, the NICU, the ER. We were chronically understaffed. Midday, the house supervisor would tell us we needed to send someone home and put them on call because of "productivity." It's called "staffing by numbers." It ignores the acuity of patients and leads to understaffing for patients who need intensive monitoring or who are undergoing lengthy, complex procedures like a bedside bronchoscopy or tracheostomy. Nurses who were sent home lost pay. It felt like the hospital was entering a new season: colder, austere. That happens sometimes. Managers leave. You have an interim for a while, even for a few years. Nurses leave. Albuquerque is a neighborhood of hospitals. A certain number of nurses are always coming and going in every hospital. Leave, come back years later. Make the round of hospitals like barhopping. It's hard to burn a bridge. The grass may not be greener, but there's grass everywhere. Hospice, home health, schools, clinics, urgent care. Nursing homes. Prisons. The quality of care declines. It's a cycle you've lived through. Then the season changes and things get better. The cheap IV kits, the floating, the understaffing made work more difficult. It was challenging but it didn't seem unfamiliar.

Then came the deaths.

8

I'm Sorry

It's four o'clock. I'm getting a transfer from Med-Surg. I look at her chart before they bring her. Camilla Diaz, 54 years old. An elective hysterectomy from Socorro. Diagnosed with uterine fibroids. Heavy menstrual bleeding. Pain. They did the surgery laparoscopically. Sandoval was the doc. Post-Op day 1. They're in the unit. The nurse is someone I don't know. A tech is helping her push the stretcher. Behind them are a young man and a woman who look to be in their early 30s. The patient's children. She's sitting straight up in the bed like she's a rodeo queen on a float during the parade they have in Santa Fe the day before the rodeo opens. Her eyes are wide. She's staring at me. We line up the stretcher and the bed. She scoots over by herself with no help. She almost seems excited. Gavin and Kristen hook her up while I step out of the room to get report from the nurse. She tells me they called a REACT on her at four in the morning for hypotension. A REACT is an overhead page initiated by a floor nurse that summons the ICU charge nurse to the bedside to assess a patient. They didn't transfer her to the ICU. At eight o'clock in the morning she was still hypotensive. They didn't call a REACT. The surgeon's at Westside. He's managing her on his own. There's no hospitalist on the case. She's in severe pain but they're not giving pain meds because she's hypotensive. They're not giving her fluid because they don't want to overload her. The nurse is young, maybe mid-20s. She has an oval face. Small gold hoop earrings. A rose tattoo on her wrist. She doesn't have any notes. The patient's pressure at noon was 82/54. The nurse didn't call the surgeon until three o'clock and he said to transfer her to the ICU. She hasn't voided since ten o'clock. She only has one IV. I ask the nurse what the patient's Is and Os are, labs. She doesn't know. I'm thinking she doesn't know anything and they're not treating her, so I tell her OK, thanks. We'll get her into the ICU and figure it out. I ask Maria, the unit secretary, to call the hospitalist and tell him she's here and he needs to come. Gavin and Kristen have her all settled. "What do you need?" Gavin asks. I tell him I need another line. I tell Kristen I'm going to need a Foley. I'll get the order from the doc. A rainbow of labs. There are things you need that you know they'll order so you just go ahead and do them. She's on the monitor. Her heart rate is 124. Her pressure is 81/52. She's watching me. She's Hispanic. Rich black hair. She's pale. There's a sheen of perspiration on her forehead. A dark crescent of moisture at the top of her hospital gown that clings to her chest. Her kids are in the room, cowering in the corner, close to each other. Been here all night. I try to imagine what these hours have been like for them. When I go to the bed she grabs my hand. I ask her where her pain is. She puts the palm of her other hand on her stomach. Her face tightens. I lift her gown. There are three laparoscopic incision sites covered with Dermabond, a translucent window of glue. They're less than an inch long. They're the way in and the way out. They go in, cut the uterus into pieces and take it out through the incisions. I know why she seems so excited. Somewhere she knows something has gone wrong. She thinks we can save her. Emmanuel Levinas developed a philosophy of the face. He says the face of the Other calls to us. "The face speaks. It is a silent and imperative language. It says: 'Do not leave me in solitude. Do not kill me.'" Her face was saying, "Save me."[1]

Pain is the check-engine light of medicine. You have to think they nicked something. It can happen from the needle they use to flow gas, usually carbon dioxide, into the stomach. It expands the abdomen so they have space to see and manipulate the instruments. Or from the trocar. The trocar is a hollow tube you pass cameras and instruments through. It's sharp, pointed like an awl. Postoperative pain, tachycardia, and fever should make you suspicious for a perforation. The intestines aren't sterile. There's fecal matter, bacteria. Bacteria spills into areas that are sterile—the blood, liver, kidneys. It's called bacterial translocation. I'm thinking of the differential diagnosis: Did she perforate? Is she bleeding? Is she going septic? No urine output. She needs fluid. I squeeze her hand back. "I'm going to help you. I'm going to give you some pain medication." The hospitalist comes, sees her, writes orders. He calls the surgeon, who says he'll be there when he finishes at Westside. We give her a liter bolus of normal saline and start her on Lactated Ringers at 150 an hour. Put a Foley in. Draw two sets of blood cultures. Send labs off. Start her on Zosyn and Bactrim, two broad-spectrum antibiotics. Order a KUB—a kidney, ureter, and bladder X-ray—to look for air in her stomach. I tell the son and daughter our plan—the tests we're going to do, how we're going to treat her pain—so they know the road ahead.

I see Leanna in the unit. The herald of nights. Shift change. She's always the first to arrive. She usually brings something she baked. Then Mateo with Sarah. The respiratory therapists round together to sign off. Mateo has a walrus mustache. He wears a white coat. When Gavin sees him, Gavin calls out, "Primo." Cousin. They exchange books. I hear Mateo say, "You have to get through the first part. Something about the Russian Revolution." From Maria's phone I hear lyrics from the song she plays at the end of the shift—"Tennessee Whiskey" by Chris Stapleton. No surgeon yet. I look into the patient's room. Those wide, staring eyes are closed. The children in chairs, on their phones, texting. From falling down a mountain, they found a ledge to rest on.

I'm off for three days. When I go back, there's a different patient in the room. I found out she crashed that night, was intubated, was on three pressors. The next afternoon, less than 24 hours after she came to the ICU, she coded and died.

We have a small break room next to the nurses' station. It has a round table with two chairs, a standing refrigerator, a coffee machine, a microwave, a counter-top refrigerator with Jello, yogurt, and juices for the patients. On the wall above the table is a magnetic bulletin board. It's usually cluttered with messages from administration, a list of Daisy Award nominees, the cafeteria menu for the week. The upper left corner is Gavin's. He writes things. A quotation. A thought. A song lyric. "It's never too late to be what you might have been."—George Eliot. When Bob Dylan won the Nobel Prize in Literature, Gavin changed the lyrics from "Tangled Up in Blue" to, "She opened up a book of poems, / And handed it to me, / Written by an American poet, / From the twentieth century." He writes something new every week. This week it's "Day one or one day. You decide." In the lower right corner is a card. The card is a scene, a winding country road running through a green valley that disappears into distant hills. The setting sun is a soft glow behind thin clouds. Over the scene, from the sky down to the road, is written, "Some People Go the Extra Mile." You open the card and it says, "THANKS For Being one of them." The handwriting is in print.

> To the ICU staff that took care of my beloved mother Camilla Diaz. I know in my heart you all did everything to save her but she was very sick and I'm grateful. Maggie RN & Ramona RN who I spoke with were just amazing ladies always making sure my family with my mother were

cared for as well as taking the time to speak with me & letting me know they were available anytime. We are utterly and eternally grateful for you two. We will always remember the great care you gave. On a personal note to me an RN is one of the hardest professions in this world, & Maggie/Ramona you guys are doing the RN title great service. Thank you for everything! Daughter Angelique Son Albert & Family!

In June 1598, Juan de Oñate led a group of Spanish settlers through the Jornada del Muerto (Route of the Dead Man), a 100-mile arid desert trail that ended at the pueblo of Teypana. As the Spaniards emerged from the desert, Piro Indians of the pueblo gave them food and water. The Spaniards renamed the pueblo Socorro, which means "help" or "aid." Socorro is 75 miles south of Albuquerque down I-25. It's 20 miles north of the Bosque del Apache National Wildlife Refuge, named for the Apache tribes that camped in the forests along the Rio Grande. The refuge was established in 1939 to provide a stopover site for migrating waterfowl and wintering grounds for sandhill cranes. From early November to mid-February over 10,000 sandhill cranes winter in the Bosque and over 20,000 Ross's and snow geese stop on their migration south. An annual "festival of the cranes" is held the weekend before Thanksgiving. Visitors arrive before dawn to see thousands of cranes and geese milling on the water. As the sun rises, the flocks rise in a cacophony of sound and wing, the snow geese first, followed by the sandhill cranes.

I imagine the family leaving early. The son driving. The mother riding shotgun. The daughter in the back. They talk. She raised them alone for many years and they're close. They pass the exit to the Albuquerque International Sunport. They take the Montgomery exit and drive east. The daughter says, "Look at the mountains." The bare western wall of the Sandias is blurry in a morning haze like someone waking. The hospital appears on their left. The mother takes a deep breath. The daughter says, "It's OK,

Mom," and puts her hand on her shoulder. Park. Front door. Check in. Pre-op. Surgery. Laparoscopic hysterectomies are usually outpatient surgeries. Post-anesthesia care unit for a few hours. Out in a wheelchair. In the evening light, the Sandias are the watermelon color the Spanish named them for. Back down I-25. But they keep her. Why? Was it pain? Blood pressure? I remember her face, looking, despite fear and pain, lovely, open, expressive, looking at me with hope that she was being brought to a place where she would be saved. Thinking maybe one night and then back to Socorro, back to her life.

In December 2004, Donald Berwick, president and CEO of the Institute for Healthcare Improvement, during his keynote address at the institute's 16th Annual National Forum on Quality Improvement in Health Care in Orlando, Florida, announced the first-ever national campaign to save 100,000 lives in the next 18 months, and every year thereafter, in US hospitals.[2] The 100,000 Lives Campaign would ask thousands of hospitals across the country to make a commitment to implement changes that have been proved to prevent avoidable deaths. To endorse this campaign, leaders of several organizations—including the American Medical Association, the American Nurses Association, and the Joint Commission on Accreditation of Healthcare Organizations—joined Berwick on-stage.

One of the Institute for Healthcare Improvement's recommendations was rapid-response teams (RRTs). Patients exhibit signs and symptoms of deterioration for several hours before a cardiac or respiratory arrest. Changes in heart rate, respiratory rate, blood pressure, mental status, urine output, and level of pain can portend a life-threatening event. RRTs bring critical care expertise to the bedside. A code blue is a response to a patient already in cardiac arrest. The goal of an RRT is to intervene upstream from a potential code, before deterioration turns into crisis. The goal is to respond to a spark before it becomes a forest fire. RRTs have names like STAR or STAT. The RRT at Women's is called REACT, Response Emergency Assessment Crisis Team. It's the ICU charge nurse, the ICU respiratory therapist, the house supervisor, and the primary nurse caring for the patient. We assess the patient, diagnose, maybe make an initial intervention like improved IV access, respiratory support, diagnostic testing—labs or an EKG. We decide if the patient should be transferred to the ICU, have their care remain with the primary physician, or have their treatment plan revised. If we don't transfer them, we go back and check on them later in the shift. We don't forget about them.

Laura was the night ICU charge. She went to the REACT. She doesn't have a lot of critical care experience. She's new at charge. The patient should have come to the ICU the previous night. We had beds. She needed intensive care monitoring. Vital signs, Is and Os every hour. They should have called another REACT in the morning when she was still hypotensive. Hours and hours went by as she deteriorated. On Med-Surg, the techs do the vital signs and then enter them manually into the electronic medical record. They might have to do vital signs on 15 patients. They write them on a piece of paper and then record them all at once. Time goes by before they're recorded and more time until the nurse looks at them in the computer. The nurse doesn't call the surgeon until late afternoon. Laura didn't tell us in her report that there had been a REACT that night.

She was septic. There are three stages: sepsis, severe sepsis, septic shock. The risk of death from sepsis is as high as 30%, for severe sepsis 50%, for septic shock 80%. Approximately 1,400 people die from sepsis every day throughout the world. The Surviving Sepsis Campaign is a global initiative to reduce mortality from sepsis.[3] It began in 2009 and has developed International Guidelines for Management of Sepsis and Septic Shock. The fifth iteration of the guidelines was published in October 2021 with 93 recommendations for the management of sepsis. Within the first three hours of suspected sepsis, you need to get a white blood cell count, a serum lactate, and blood cultures and start antibiotics. The chance of sepsis progressing to septic shock and death increases by 4% to 9% every hour treatment is delayed. An increased risk of death is already present by the second hour after the onset of hypotension.

RRTs are successful when they're called earlier and more often and when it is ensured that, when they get there, they always do the right thing. At the REACT, it was like a gate opened to the ICU and they didn't do the right thing and the gate closed.

In a 1975 article R. Adams Cowley wrote, "The first hour after injury will largely determine a critically injured person's chances for survival." He called this time the "Golden Hour." The underlying tenet is that in the period of 60 minutes or less following traumatic injury, there is the highest likelihood that prompt medical and surgical treatment will prevent death.[4]

There's a golden hour in the ICU. Years ago, nurses didn't carry stethoscopes, auscultate the lungs, identify heart sounds. There was no CPR, no cardiac defibrillation, no resuscitation. Now nurses do the rule of nines on burn patients to determine fluid replacement, recognize life-threatening arrhythmias, call codes, titrate powerful vasoactive drugs that can restore and maintain hemodynamic stability. The intensive care is intensive nursing care. If you're free-falling into death, we can save you. If you come to us in time.

Daniel Chambliss writes, "In hospitals, as a normal part of the routine, people suffer and die." Death is not unexpected. Only combat forces share this feature. Nurses adapt to pain and death. It's what separates them from the rest of us. Sociologists try to see how hospitals resemble other organizations, "but we should not make a premature leap to commonalities before appreciating the unique features of hospitals that make a nurse's task so different from that of a teacher, a businessman, or a bureaucrat."[5]

Most patients who die in a hospital die in the ICU. We do adapt to death. Most of the time it's not a surprise. Sometimes the patient is so sick, death is inevitable. You can see it on the horizon, every day getting closer. Maybe they've already coded once. Or they die after weeks where they've fought for their life and you've done all you could and everyone knows it's the end of the day. But she shouldn't have died. She didn't come to us intubated, unresponsive. She came a fresh post-op, awake, wide-eyed, hopeful.

It felt more tragic than other deaths, so preventable. There were so many opportunities to recognize what was wrong, intervene, stabilize her. So many errors of judgment, wrong decisions. If the surgeon doesn't want to transfer her to the ICU and you think she should be there, you can go up the chain of command: charge nurse, house supervisor, chief nursing officer, medical director. No one did that. It felt like her death indicated that something was wrong, something was broken. The chief nursing officer was in her office. I told her what happened. How the REACT was called but she wasn't transferred to the ICU. That we should try to find out what happened at the REACT. Why they made the decision not to transfer her. Why the next shift didn't call a REACT when she hadn't improved. I said it was a never event. She quickly said it wasn't a never event. She said she would talk to the charge nurses.

The Leapfrog Group, founded in 2000, is the nation's premier advocate of transparency in health care. Its goal is to help employers and other health-care consumers choose which hospital will provide care for their employees by collecting, analyzing, and publishing data on the quality, affordability, and safety of American hospitals. Leapfrog rates hospitals through the Leapfrog Hospital Survey and the Leapfrog Hospital Safety Grade. Hospitals voluntarily submit data through the survey. In 2019 and 2020, over 2,300 hospitals submitted a Leapfrog Hospital Survey. The Leapfrog Hospital Safety Grade assigns letter grades, A, B, C, D, or F, to hospitals based on their record of patient safety.

In 2007, the year after the National Quality Forum released its list of never events, Leapfrog chose to support the work of the forum by asking hospitals in the Leapfrog Hospital Survey about their process for handling never events. Leapfrog asked hospitals to commit to five actions if a never event occurs within their facility: (1) apologize to the patient, (2) report the event, (3) perform a root cause analysis, (4) waive costs directly related to the event, and (5) provide a copy of the hospital's policy on never events to patients upon request. The National Quality Forum says when discussing a never event with a patient or family member, the physician must deliver a sincere apology that includes the word "sorry."

Twenty-nine states have laws that make expressions of sympathy following an accident or error inadmissible in civil court as evidence to prove liability. Referred to as "I'm sorry" laws, the legislation encourages full disclosure of mistakes or errors by eliminating the physician's and the hospital's fear that their admissions will be used against them in a court of law. New Mexico is one of 12 states that does not have an "I'm sorry" law and allows the admission of sympathetic statements as evidence of malpractice.

There are seven categories of never events. Section 1 is Surgical or Invasive Procedure Events. Section 1E is an intraoperative or immediately postoperative death in an American Society of Anesthesiologists (ASA) Class 1 patient. An ASA Class 1 patient is a normal healthy patient.

She was a normal healthy patient. Maggie was her nurse the day she died. She's a good nurse. I can see her in the room. Asking the physician what he wants for a second and a third pressor in case she needs it. Titrating drips. Drawing blood for arterial blood gas tests. She has the crash cart just outside the room in case the patient codes. She has the defibrillator pads on the patient's chest to be ready. She never leaves the room. The children are in chairs. Maggie tells them everything she's doing. Explains the ventilator to them. Shows them the arterial blood gas analysis results.

Answers all their questions. I can see why they said they would be utterly and eternally grateful. They saw someone doing all they could to save their mother's life. What they didn't see were the mistakes, the negligence, the failures that came before.

It wasn't a never event. She wasn't a 1E patient. She didn't die immediately after surgery. She died more than 24 hours later. But someone should have said, "I'm sorry."

9

We Know Their Names

He was on Med-Surg in a room just across from the door to the ICU. There was always a small crowd outside his room. One day, his nurse called the ICU and asked if someone was free to put an IV in him. I was caught up. He was a white-haired, somewhat heavy guy sitting up in bed. I introduced myself. His name was Philip Garrett. He smiled and said, "They say you're the expert." "Well now you've jinxed me," I said. I put a tourniquet on his right arm, tricked out an antecubital vein, and slid an 18 gauge in. "Did you get it?" he asked. "I did." "I guess they were right," he laughed. As I walked by the small crowd, a woman holding her iPhone to her ear looked at me and quietly mouthed, "Thank you."

It's three days later. Denise, the house supervisor, comes into the ICU and says to me, "Can you come check on a guy for me? They've been calling Garcia all day. He's at LMC." Most of the hospitalists are in-house, from Lovelace Medical Group. But some of them are from DaVita, an outside group the hospital also contracts with. Garcia is DaVita. The patient is Philip Garrett. I walk by the same small crowd. His eyes are closed, his head to the side, his skin pale. He's on oxygen. The pronged nasal cannula is attached to a flowmeter behind the bed. I say his name, "Mr. Garrett." No response. I feel for his radial pulse. It's weak. His skin is cool, clammy. His abdomen is distended and rigid. There are more people in the room. The house supervisor. The Med-Surg charge. Some floor nurses. I ask who his nurse is. A young nurse raises her hand at chest level.

"What's he in for?"

"Colitis."

Dr. Perez comes in the room. He's the hospitalist today. He's a fairly new doc. He's from Manhattan. He hasn't been at Lovelace Women's Hospital long. Some of them come to New Mexico to work off their medical school loans like we're a third-world country. One day he said to me, "You look like someone who likes Bob Dylan." Dylan was coming to the KiMo Theater in Albuquerque and he had tickets. He told me he went to Coachella. That Beyoncé played the same show both weekends. That he saw Billy Joel at Madison Square Garden. He went to medical school in Cuba. Has a daughter there. He's thinking of going to Florida to be near her.

Mr. Garrett is not his patient. He doesn't have to be here. I look at him. I can't make the decision to transfer a patient on my own. He'll be dead by midnight. "He's DaVita's. Garcia's at LMC. He needs to go to the ICU." We're East Coast guys. I feel like he knows me. Knows I'm a good nurse. He nods twice.

We're in the ICU but we have no orders. The ICU is said to be eleven hours of boredom and one hour of terror. I ask Maria to call Garcia. We get him on the ICU bed. He's a dead lift. His nurse gives me report in the room. We're hooking him up. His pressure is 78/40. She says he came in a week ago with abdominal pain. Diagnosed with colitis. The plan was medical management. I ask her what happened today. She says he had more abdominal pain. She called the doctor and he said he would be in later.

"When did his level of consciousness change?"

She looked at me.

"He's unresponsive. I put an IV in him three days ago. He was awake and alert."

Gavin draws blood for an arterial blood gas analysis and Sarah runs it right away on a portable machine she has with her. His pH is 7.20. His oxygen is 58, carbon dioxide 51. Garcia's on the phone. I tell him we brought the patient to the ICU. That he's unresponsive, hypotensive. I tell him the gas. That he needs to be intubated. He says he'll call the ER. "Start him on an epi drip." A patient on a ventilator is managed by our pulmonologist. I tell him I need to consult Dr. O'Neill. Maria gets O'Neill on the phone. He gives me vent settings. Start him on Levophed. Normal saline bolus on a pressure bag. Labs. Two sets of blood cultures. Flagyl and Zosyn q 8, first dose now. Fifty grams of albumin. Two amps of bicarb. A venous blood gas analysis after intubation. "Foley, NG?" I'm putting Garcia on the backburner. He didn't come.

The ER doctor walks in the room with a young woman behind him. He has the kind of swagger ER docs can have, but that's OK, he's going to help us.

"You need somebody intubated?"

"What do you want?"

"Etomidate. Versed."

He has no problem getting the tube in.

"Anything else you need?"

"A central line?"

"They like putting it in the neck, I like the groin."

"The groin's fine."

The young woman is standing against the wall. She looks terrified.

"Who are you?"

"His scribe."

He opened the doors we needed. We need to get inside the body. When you're dying, we need what we call access: We need to get into your lungs, your veins, your bladder. Take over your body like somebody at Apple Support takes over your computer.

I let the family in two at a time. It's always the same, the way their breath catches and they step back like when you open the door of a hot oven. It must be a shock going from seeing him last week sitting in bed, talking, to seeing him now, with the endotracheal tube coming out of his mouth like the tongue in that movie *Alien*, attached to a machine the size of a stove.

The surgeon is here. He looks at the patient's abdomen. Asks me what meds he's on. When he leaves, he says to me, "We'll take him around two." The anesthesiologist and the operating room nurse come for him at two thirty. The middle of the room is suddenly empty, like when you take out the pit of an avocado. I look at his chart. History of hypertension and coronary disease. Came in with abdominal pain and bloody diarrhea. Diagnosed with colitis. The plan was supportive measures and medical management, empiric antibiotic, a liquid diet.

We call it dead gut. Blood flow to the bowel stops. The entire wall of the bowel can die. It's called a transmural infarction, a surgical emergency. The mortality rate is 80%–100% if you don't get to surgery within 24 hours from the onset of symptoms. The only treatment is immediate removal of the dead bowel segment.

He comes back just before six. They did a total colectomy, gave him an ileostomy.

For the next two weeks, every day I worked, he was my assignment. He went into septic shock. Maxed on pressors. His kidneys failed. They put a catheter into his subclavian vein for hemodialysis. When someone is intubated, we put the work of breathing—the workload—onto the machine. As the patient improves, we gradually shift the workload back to the patient. It's called weaning. We couldn't wean him. His ventilator settings remained high. Oxygen at 100%.

It's the beginning of the third week. We're having a family meeting in the waiting room just outside the ICU. It's a small room, two couches and a chair. A wall TV. I know them all pretty well. They come at different times of the day. Before work. Lunch breaks. After work. Sit for hours in the chairs. Two weeks is a long time. It's like you're passengers on a cruise ship together. See each other on the deck. In the dining hall. Get to know each other. They ask questions. If they're doing dialysis. Whether they've been able to come down on the vent. Whether he has a fever. There's just so much to ask, and after a while they'll ask about you. How long you've been a nurse. Where you're from. How long you've been in New Mexico. The woman outside Mr. Garrett's room who said "thank you" after I put in the IV turned out to be his daughter Pam. She comes in a lot. Sometimes with others, the patient's wife, her own son and daughter; sometimes alone. Different times of the day. She told me stories about her father. How he wasn't able to go to college. How he built a successful business and made sure all his kids went to college. How he loved to hike and when he was young once climbed Mt. Rainier. She told me they were estranged for years. She was a singer. She wanted to study music. He didn't think that was practical. She went to Oberlin. It came between them. She's the music director at Sagebrush Church in the North Valley. Things changed when she had her own kids. He was a great grandfather. But they were lost years.

The family is his wife, Pam and another daughter, a son, spouses. In the family meeting, I stand behind O'Neill. He says the patient's kidneys weren't "happy." That they haven't been able to lower the ventilator settings. Then he talks about a tracheostomy and a percutaneous endoscopic gastrostomy (PEG) and transfer to a long-term care nursing facility. In a PEG, they make an incision into the abdominal wall and put a flexible feeding tube directly into the stomach. That's how you feed them, give them fluids and medications. It's usually for someone who's unconscious, in a coma, who will never wake up. When someone is on a ventilator, a tube—the endotracheal tube—is inserted to just above the carina, a ridge of cartilage at the lower end of the trachea above the lungs. The tube is nine inches long. For patients who can't breathe on their own and are facing long-term mechanical ventilation, they do a tracheostomy. They make a small incision in the neck and place a shorter tube, about four inches long, into the trachea. It's more comfortable. It's easier to do oral care. Trach and PEG is what you do when there's no more to be done. "To warehouse" a patient is hospital slang. It means sending patients somewhere, usually a nursing home, where they get little or no medical care. Sometimes in rounds, case management will let slip that someone is going to be warehoused the next day. Trach and PEG is what you get before you go to the warehouse.

O'Neill leaves. I stay. Pam looks up at me and asks, "What do you think, Jim?" I think the thing O'Neill didn't say, that I think they want, but don't know how to say: it's time to stop.

I was standing in the doorway facing them, my back to Med-Surg. Kristen once said that I have speeches. She meant it in a kind way. I do. There are things I say every time, not because I came up with them myself but because, early on in the Neuro ICU at the University of New Mexico Hospital, there was so much death and I would have to talk with families about withdrawing care, and I was new and didn't know what to say, and over time I learned what they were thinking, what they were afraid of, what they wanted to happen. I learned what to say from that. I sometimes think it may be me talking, but it's a memory of those voices I heard years ago when I was new.

"I think we have to ask ourselves what he would want. About quality of life. Would he want to be in a long-term care facility on a ventilator? On dialysis. Never wake up. Never be able to feed himself." Some of them shake their head. A few say, "He wouldn't want that."

"We've treated him every day as if one day he'll walk out of the ICU. That's been our hope. But at some point, you realize he's not getting better. I think he's actively dying." Families will say they don't want to be the ones to make the decision, to "pull the plug." They don't want to live with that. I tell them what I believe. I say that they shouldn't think of it as their decision, as them deciding to let him die. That it's the patient's decision. The patient is telling us that his life has come to an end, and we have to accept that decision.

"Medicine man" is an Anglicized term for a Native American healer. The Navajo word is *haatali*, or "singer." The singer comes to where the sick person is and does a healing ceremony. He'll bring a medicine pouch—*jish* in Navajo—with sacred objects that have spiritual or supernatural power: herbs, rattles, fetishes, small pottery bowls, whistles, shells, feathers, pouches of sacred pollen. He'll chant. My first year in nursing at St. Joe's, we had a Navajo patient who was dying. Days went by. The family was there. The waiting was hard. It was as if there was something stopping him. Something in the way. The singer came. He didn't stay very long. A half an hour after he left, the patient died. I asked his nurse what the singer did. She said he opened a window so his spirit could leave.

Physicians almost never talk about withdrawing care. They never say how it's actually done. Sometimes you have to open a window so the family can see the way out, how it can end.

I tell them how it would end. They would be in the room. I would ask them to step outside into the hall. Pull the curtain. We would take out the endotracheal tube. I would stop all the drips. They would come back in. They could all be with him. We would give him medication so he wouldn't suffer. He would die peacefully, without fear. I tell them there are things we can do here in the ICU that can't be done if he leaves here, if he's in a nursing home, that here they have a choice they won't have again. They ask questions: "We could be with him?" "He wouldn't suffer?" I leave them to talk among themselves.

I'm in his room next to the bed pushing a med when Pam comes in alone. She stands next to me. She's quiet. "Tomorrow morning," she says softly. "We'd like to do it tomorrow morning."

I call O'Neill to tell him they want to withdraw in the morning. He's surprised. He asks me what made them come to that decision. I tell him that after he left, they stayed and talked among themselves. He says he'll write orders.

That the patient won't suffer is a promise. Withdrawing care is like firing a pot. You get one shot at it. It will be the last image families will have. The last moments of life. You can't have the patient awake, gasping for air, struggling. Physicians differ in what they'll prescribe for the end. O'Neill's frugal. I know what he'll order. Morphine and Ativan 2–4 mg every hour. That's not enough. His partner is the opposite. He'll write morphine and Ativan 5–20 mg every 30 minutes and say to me, "Give him lots of drugs." Even though O'Neill is the primary, writing all the orders, DaVita is still on the case. It's a different hospitalist. Martinez. She's a good doctor. If I have one of her patients, she'll find me in the unit so we can go into the room together. After she writes orders, she'll call me over and tell me what the plan is. She does rounds every day, talks to whatever family is there, asks me how it's going. I call her and tell her my concern. What O'Neill would order. How it wouldn't be enough. I tell her what the other doctor would order. "Write what you want," she says, "and I'll sign it." I write morphine 5–20 mg q 30 minutes. Ativan 5–20 mg q 30 minutes. May repeat times one if necessary.

Back in the room, I go to the side of the bed. I look down at him. Tomorrow is his last day on earth. The nasogastric tube is in his right nostril. The endotracheal tube is in the left corner of his mouth. The respiratory therapists move it every day so his lips won't break down. It's secured by white tape that goes around his neck. His hair has a greasy sheen. His cheeks are covered with white stubble. Pam had told me he took great pride in his appearance, how important it was to him. He wore a suit to work every day. He was always clean-shaven.

Jason, the respiratory therapist, helps me. He untapes the endotracheal tube and holds it in place so I can shave him. We have these no-rinse shampoo caps that you microwave for a few seconds to activate. You put them on like a swimmer's cap and then massage the scalp. After, I comb his hair. So he's ready. The Spanish poet Juan Ramón Jiménez said about death, "The first night is the hardest."

In the morning, there are maybe 15 people in the room. End-of-life we let everybody in. We had changed the sheets, pillowcase. Put a clean gown on him. After a while, Pam comes out and says they're ready. I have them step outside the room. Close the curtain. Jason takes the balloon down and pulls the tube. I give the patient 20 of morphine and 10 of Ativan. Stop the pressors. Turn down the monitor so they don't stare at it. Next to the secretary's desk is a monitor the size of a smart TV that shows the cardiac rhythms of all the ICU patients and the patients in Med-Surg on telemetry. I'll watch his heart rate in the nurses' station. They come back in and gather around the bed. Some families sing, some pray, some hold hands. Sometimes they say the Lord's Prayer together. I hear voices. "I love you, Dad." "Thank you, Dad." "We're all here." I go in the room and give him another 20 of morphine even though his eyes are closed and he's still. "So he won't have any fear crossing the threshold." Pam nods. When his heart rate slows down to the 30s, I go in the room and say he'll die in two minutes. If they have final words. Death is a six-second flat line on the EKG. We call the physician to come and listen to his heart and pronounce the patient dead, but the six-second strip is the time of death. We print it. When it happens, I go into the room and tell them, "He just passed."

One road is a highway. They catch it in time, you have surgery, they do a resection, maybe a colostomy for a while. You come back to the ICU. You get off pressors. Your blood pressure holds. You make urine. Wake up. You get weaned off the ventilator. Sit up in bed, talk to your family. Start with clear liquids. The diet is advanced. Get out of bed with physical therapy. Go to rehab. Then the road takes you home. On the other road, they don't catch it. Hours go by. Bacteria is spilling into your gut. The nurse doesn't recognize it. Doesn't call a REACT. You go to surgery. They take out your colon. You're in the ICU. You get septic. Your lungs get worse. They can't wean the ventilator. You're maxed on pressors. Your kidneys fail. They start dialysis. Some days they can't do it because your pressure drops. You puff up from the fluid you can't pee out and dialysis can't pull off. It seeps into your lungs, pushes back against your heart. You develop arrhythmias. The sedation is off but you never wake up. There are rocks and debris on the highway, so you get onto a two-lane road. It turns into a one-way, then dirt. It narrows to ruts. Then there's no road. He took that road.

It was an afternoon in the unit a few days later. We were talking about Camilla Diaz's children. How kind they were. The card they wrote. Then the conversation shifted to how Pam came to the unit the day after and thanked everyone for all they did for her father. How sad it was. It was Maggie who said it. "It's a failure to rescue."

The term "failure to rescue" first appeared in a 1992 study led by Jeffrey Silber of the Center for Outcomes Research at the Children's Hospital of Philadelphia.[1] The original research was on surgical patients who developed complications and died. The term was later extended to patients with medical conditions. Failure to rescue is failure to recognize and respond to non-ICU patients experiencing complications or acute clinical deterioration and bring them back from the edge of death. The idea is that, although not every complication of medical care is preventable, health-care systems should be able to rapidly identify and treat complications when they occur. That they should not die.

Failure to rescue is strongly linked to nursing. Monitoring and surveillance are essential but distinct nursing activities. Monitoring involves observation, measurement, and recording of physiological parameters such as blood pressure, pulse, respirations, and oxygen level. Surveillance is the interpretation of that data for clinical decision-making. Surveillance is detecting changes, interpreting their clinical implications, and initiating appropriate interventions. Nurses have a pivotal role in recognizing the changes that can signal complications and intervening to prevent a cascade of events that leads to death. Failure to rescue can be failure to monitor, failure to recognize, or failure to escalate and activate a team response. In 2004, the National Quality Forum selected failure to rescue as a core measure for evaluating the performance of nursing care in acute care hospitals.

In "Failure to Rescue: An Evidence Based Glimpse," Jacy L. Henk asks how the profession of nursing could reach the point of eliminating failure-to-rescue events so that they would go into nursing textbooks as something that no longer happens.[2] An essential action is the nurturing of younger and new graduate nurses. Inexperienced nurses should be seen and treated as an investment in the future of the profession. They need to be taught how to do surveillance on their patients as well as the patients of other nurses. Citing Patricia Benner, Henk writes that nurses leave nursing school as novices and enter the profession as advanced beginners.[3] It is the responsibility of experienced, expert nurses to transform them into competent and proficient nurses.

The challenge facing advanced beginners is recognizing the concrete manifestations of clinical signs and symptoms. They strive to "see" and recognize clinical entities they have studied only theoretically: dyspnea, hypertensive crisis, refractory hypoxemia.[4] They lack sufficient practical experience to respond to and manage changing critical care situations. Consequently, they need coaching about what interventions are needed. Advanced beginners rely on their colleagues for advice as to when to give "as-needed" medications, repeat a lab, call the physician. When situations arise where advanced beginners lack confidence, they go up the clinical ladder to nurses who have greater experience and authority. The strategy of "delegating up" provides for safe patient care in situations beyond the advanced beginner's experience.[5] Delegating complex clinical observations and decisions depends on the availability of a cadre of experienced and knowledgeable nurses. The advanced beginner's progress through the stages of skill acquisition requires the precepting and situated teaching and coaching of proficient-to-expert nurses. It is an essential feature of the nursing practice environment, as Benner, Christine A. Tanner, and Catherine A. Chesla note: "When an advanced beginner asks an experienced clinician for a judgment, it is an unrepeatable teaching opportunity. All clinicians have gained their comparative judgments and wisdom similarly. It is a clinical responsibility to pass that hard-won experiential learning on to the beginning clinicians."[6]

The nursing practice environment has been defined as one of the organizational characteristics of a work setting that facilitate or constrain professional nursing practice. The Practice Environment Scale of the Nursing Work Index is an instrument that measures the nursing practice environment. It is endorsed by the National Quality Forum. The scale has five categories:

(1) Nurse participation in hospital affairs: There are career development and clinical ladder opportunities, there are opportunities for staff nurses to participate in policy

decisions, staff nurses are involved in the internal governance of the hospital (e.g., practice and policy committees), and nursing administrators consult with staff on
daily problems and procedures.

(2) Nursing foundations for quality of care: There are active
staff development or continuing education programs for
nurses, high standards of nursing care are expected by
the administration, nurses work with nurses who are
clinically competent, and there is an active quality
assurance program.

(3) Nurse manager ability, leadership, and support of nurses:
There is a supervisory staff that is supportive of the
nurses, and supervisors use mistakes as learning opportunities, not opportunities for criticism.

(4) Staffing and resource adequacy: Adequate support
services allow nurses to spend time with their patients,
there is enough time and opportunity to discuss patient
care problems with other nurses, and there are enough
registered nurses to provide quality patient care.

(5) Collegial nurse-physician relations: There is a collaborative, working relationship between nurses and physicians.

Because private equity expects to exit an investment in three
to five years, it has little concern for the viability of the company
beyond that investment horizon. The culture of work, the professional development of nurses, job satisfaction, the benefits of
retention, and the preoccupation with safety are not concerns of
private equity firms. As private equity firms increase their profits
more from financial engineering than productive activities, the
incentive to invest in workers' skills declines. The idea of labor as
a fixed asset or human capital as valuable loses force. Employees
are seen as dispensable, a variable cost to be minimized. Job destruction and intensification of work for those who remain follow

private equity acquisitions. Private equity companies cut staff, re-duce wages and benefits, and eliminate raises. Experienced workers who helped build a business, employees who have in-vested 10 or 20 years of their lives helping a company grow, can be fired with little or no notice and without a severance package.

Private equity cost-cutting targets nursing because it is the larg-est expense for hospitals, with salaries and benefits accounting for between 40% and 55% of total operating costs despite decades of research that has documented how safe staffing improves re-covery and reduces patient mortality. A principal finding of a 1996 report by the Institute of Medicine's Committee on the Adequacy of Nurse Staffing in Hospitals and Nursing Homes was the impor-tance of nurse staffing to the delivery of high-quality patient care: "Nursing is a critical factor in determining the quality of care in hospitals and the nature of patient outcomes."[7] The finding later became conceptualized as "nurse-sensitive measures," which have been defined as outcomes where evidence has linked nurs-ing interventions with patient outcomes. Patient mortality, medi-cation error, pressure injury, hospital-acquired infection, and patient fall are the most frequently examined patient outcomes. Understaffing and high nurse-patient ratios have a negative effect on patient outcomes. "Each additional patient per nurse is asso-ciated with 12% higher odds of in-hospital mortality, 7% higher odds of 60-day mortality, 7% higher odds of 60-day readmission, and longer lengths of stay."[8] A study conducted by the University of Pennsylvania School of Nursing's Center for Health Outcomes and Policy Research found that "in hospitals with high nurse-to-patient ratios, each additional patient per nurse was associated with . . . a 7% increase" in the likelihood of a failure to rescue.[9]

Ardent's view of nursing as solely an economic variable is ex-plicit in the IPO prospectus: "Our expenses depend upon the levels of salaries and benefits paid to our employees, the cost of supplies and the costs of other operating expenses."[10] The "Risk Factors" section explains,

> We compete with other healthcare providers in recruiting and retaining qualified management and support personnel responsible for the daily operations of each of our hospitals, including nurses and other non-physician healthcare professionals. In some markets, the availability of nurses and other medical support personnel has been a significant operating issue for healthcare providers. We may be required to continue to enhance wages and benefits to recruit and retain nurses and other medical support personnel or to hire more expensive temporary or contract personnel, which could increase our labor costs. . . . In addition, the states in which we operate could adopt mandatory nurse-staffing ratios or could reduce mandatory nurse staffing ratios already in place. State-mandated nurse-staffing ratios could significantly affect labor costs and have an adverse impact on revenues if we are required to limit admissions or hire additional personnel in order to meet the required ratios.
>
> Increased or ongoing labor union activity is another factor that could adversely affect our labor costs or otherwise adversely impact us. To the extent a significant portion of our employee base unionizes, it is possible our labor costs could increase materially. When negotiating collective bargaining agreements with unions, whether such agreements are renewals or first contracts, there is the possibility that strikes could occur during the negotiation process, and our continued operation during any strikes could increase our labor costs. . . .
>
> If our labor costs continue to increase, we may not be able to achieve higher payer reimbursement levels or reduce other operating expenses in a manner sufficient to offset these increased labor costs. Because substantially all of our net patient service revenue are based on reimbursement rates fixed or negotiated no less frequently than annually, our ability to pass along periodic increased labor costs is

materially constrained. Our failure to recruit and retain qualified management, nurses and other medical support personnel, or to control our labor costs, could have a material adverse effect on our financial condition and results of operations.[11]

In the years since Ventas bought Ardent, it had been as if a harrow had gone through the nursing staff at Women's, decimating it by resignations, firings, forced ousters. An exodus of managers and senior nurses—experienced but also higher salaried—left behind a staff of young, inexperienced nurses. It was as if the cottonwoods in the bosque had been cut down and only an understory of shrubs and grasses remained. There was no one to aspire to be like. No one to provide shade for growth. The nurses who were left didn't know the significance of a sign or symptom, if it was benign or a portent. They lacked the confidence to trigger a team response. The nurses who took care of Camilla Diaz and Philip Garrett were new, advanced beginners. We had lost that cadre of proficient, expert nurses for them to delegate up to, who had the experience and authority to guide them through a changing clinical situation. The innate complexity and unpredictability of patient care require professional alertness and skill in preventative, monitoring, and rectifying action not fully embodied in a new nurse. It requires a culture to develop them. In the hospital setting, the cost-cutting and workforce depletion of the private equity business model erodes the nursing practice environment and puts patients at risk.

The ability to rescue patients is a nursing quality indicator, but it also reflects the resources, preparedness, and response of the hospital system. Its resiliency. From a high-reliability organization perspective, organizational resilience is based on the belief that the unexpected is inevitable; no amount of planning and anticipation will prevent all complications. Resilient teams maintain a continual awareness of the potential for things to go wrong. They collaborate, share information about the clinical situation. They continually scan for potential problems, recognize changes in a patient's condition, react quickly to mitigate problems that arise, often before they fully understand the complete nature of the problem.

When he announced the 100,000 Lives Campaign in 2004, Dr. Berwick said, "The names of the patients whose lives we save can never be known. Our contribution will be what did not happen to them. And, though they are unknown, we will know that mothers and fathers are at graduations and weddings they would have missed, and that grandchildren will know grandparents they might never have known, and holidays will be taken, and work completed, and books read, and symphonies heard, and gardens tended that, without our work, would never have been."[12]

Women's Hospital had lost its resiliency. We should have saved them but we didn't. We know their names. We know what happened to them. We know all the things they'll miss.

10

The Five Whys

It's just after noon. Gavin tells me I'm getting a patient from the ER, Gloria Baca. The protocol at Lovelace Women's Hospital for transferring a patient to the ICU is for the ER to call and ask if they can bring the patient. You tell them yes or no. You might need to go to CT. You might be getting ready to intubate someone. Is it safe to bring them? During a spacewalk, astronauts keep themselves connected to the space station with at least one tether clipped to their suit using locking metal hooks. Traveling from the ER to the ICU is like a spacewalk. You leave the safety of the spaceship. You have to be sure they're tethered. That there's a nurse, a transport person, a respiratory therapist. That they're on a monitor. That the journey is expeditious. When they arrive in the unit, the ICU staff transfers the patient to the ICU bed, connects them up to the monitor, gets a set of vital signs. The spacewalk is over. The ER nurse gives report to the ICU nurse outside the room.

Just moments after Gavin tells me, the ICU doors open. The chief nursing officer (CNO) and the house supervisor are pushing a patient on a stretcher. The CNO isn't in scrubs. She's wearing a blouse, a skirt, heels. The house supervisor is in scrubs. Neither one has a stethoscope. It's the ER admission. At the same time, Maria tells me the ER nurse in on the line to give report. Right away everything feels wrong. Protocol breached. The tether broken.

The nurse on the phone is the ER educator. She tells me that she doesn't know much about the patient because the two nurses who had been taking care of her gave report and left; she had only had her for a little while.

I go into the room. The patient is on the monitor, but the blood pressure didn't register. It timed out without a reading. No numbers. It's cycling again. You can hear the whirring sound. It times out again with no blood pressure recording. Gavin puts two fingers on her neck where the carotid artery flows. A few seconds. "I'm not getting a pulse." I look up at the monitor and see a rhythm scrolling across the screen. I look at her. Her eyes are closed. Her chest isn't moving. Gavin says, "I think we should start CPR," and begins compressions. I say, "She's in PEA [pulseless electrical activity]." Kristen tells Maria to call a code blue and goes for the crash cart. I see one of the hospitalists in the nurses' station and ask him to come into the room because we're going to run a code. We need a doctor present during a code although we all know what to do. We don't call codes and then wait for the doctor to show up. Physicians arrive at codes already going. We need them to tell us to do what we're already doing. I look to see what IVs are hanging and see a bag of Levophed that's dry. Next to it is a full, unspiked bag. I follow the line and see it's not attached to the patient. The pump is on pause. The Levophed is programmed mcg/kg/min. I spike the bag, connect the tubing, change it to mcg/min, and put it at 20. We begin the code at 12:40 p.m. We give two milligrams of epinephrine and one amp of sodium bicarb. At 13:13, we have a carotid pulse and a measured blood pressure and end the code. After the code, we intubate her.

The CNO is in the nurses' station. I ask her why the ER nurse didn't bring her up. She says the ER was full and they needed to "decompress" it, so she and the house supervisor decided they would just bring her up. She doesn't say anything when I tell her the Levophed wasn't running.

In the heart, electricity precedes pumping. The sinoatrial node is a crescent-shaped group of cells in the wall of the right atrium. It's the heart's pacemaker. It sends an electrical impulse that moves through the heart muscle and causes it to contract. The rhythm you see on the monitor has upward deflections called waves. The first wave is the P wave. It represents muscle contraction in the atria. The next wave is called the QRS complex. The electrical impulse causes the ventricles to contract and eject blood from the heart.

PEA is pulseless electrical activity. In PEA there is an organized rhythm on the monitor. P wave, QRS wave, but there's no muscle contraction. No blood flow from the heart. No pulse. Asystole is a flatline EKG with no electrical activity on the monitor. Asystole is cardiac arrest. PEA is not cardiac arrest, but it's deep into the dying process that begins with failure of the brain or the lungs. As the person enters death, the heart continues to pump until the oxygen and metabolic substrates necessary for it to function are depleted. Blood pressure drops, the heart rate slows, the pulse is lost. The loss of pulse is the initiation of PEA. Electrical activity continues but the heart no longer pumps. Then PEA becomes asystole. The heart is the last organ to fail. Two factors determine the potential for survival by resuscitation: the underlying process that is leading to death, and the length of time in the dying process when efforts to reverse it are initiated.

The ER is on the first floor in the back of the hospital. As in all ERs, the door is locked. Inside the ER there's a round metal button on the wall the size of a dinner plate that you push to open the door to a hallway that goes to the hospital lobby. The door opens slowly. It's about 80 to 90 feet to the elevators. Just before the elevators, you pause at an intersection with a hall that goes to the lab and an exit door to the back parking lot in one direction and to Pharmacy, MRI, and Central Supply in the other. There are only two elevators. It usually takes two to three minutes for an elevator to come. The elevators are small, so it takes time to fit in the bed, the pumps. The doors can close while you're getting in and you have to push them open again. The elevator opens on Med-Surg. The ICU is to your left about 30 feet away. You swipe your badge to get in. It can take up to 10 minutes to go from the ER to the ICU, get transferred to an ICU bed, and get placed on the monitor. In the ER, the Levophed was maintaining her blood pressure. At some point in the journey from the ER to the ICU, with the Levophed not infusing, her blood pressure falls. Oxygen delivery drops. The heart slows. The pulse is lost. The reversible period following cessation of pulse is referred to as "clinical death" and the irreversible as "biological death." She left the ER alive and arrived in the ICU clinically dead.

The CNO and the house supervisor aren't clinical nurses. They don't take care of patients. They don't manage drips. In the ICU, if someone is critically ill and we have to travel to MRI or CT, before we leave the unit, we call them and tell them we're on our way, that we need oxygen, suction. We want the room to be empty. We don't want someone to be on the table. Before we leave, we'll have someone get the elevator and hold the door open so we don't have to wait. We want green lights the whole way.

Patients on ventilators are sedated. We use a continuous infusion of propofol. It's a white liquid. It's known as the "milk of amnesia." Every morning we turn it off. We call it a "sedation vacation." It's for a neurological assessment; to see if they wake up, react appropriately to stimuli, if they can move all their extremities. There can be silent strokes. The next morning, I turned off the propofol at eight o'clock. Hours passed. Noon. Four o'clock. She never responded.

Anoxic brain injury occurs when the brain is deprived of oxygen. Brain cells without enough oxygen will start to die after four minutes. Severe anoxia can lead to coma. A week after she was admitted to the ICU, comatose, in multiple organ failure, the family withdrew support and she died.

The following week, I was working and the director of quality called the unit to speak to me. She asked me if I thought that the Levophed being off was the precipitating cause or a factor in the demise of the patient. "The precipitating cause," I said.

The movement of patients through a hospital is called patient flow. Patients are transferred from the ER to the ICU. From the ICU to Med-Surg. Within that, they'll go to the operating room and back. To the GI lab for an esophagogastroduodenoscopy. To radiology for films, cardiac stress tests. The transfer of essential information and the responsibility for care of the patient from one health-care provider to another is known as a handoff. It links the patient to the next provider like a carabiner. It's estimated that a typical teaching hospital may have more than 4,000 handoffs every day.

A handoff is meant to ensure continuity and safety of care, but it has the potential for harm. In 2001, the Institute of Medicine reported that inadequate handoffs are "where safety often fails first."[1] Handoffs can result in a progressive loss of information known as funneling; information is missed, forgotten, not conveyed. It can lead to medication error, delay of treatment, morbidity. Two-thirds of all sentinel events are related to communication errors, over half of which involve handoff failures.

In 2006, the Joint Commission established a National Patient Safety Goal that addressed handoff communication. Hospitals were to "implement a standardized approach to 'handoff' communications."[2] Joint Commission surveyors would want to see that the organization has a defined process for what information needs to be communicated and how it will be communicated. They will want to know that those expectations have been communicated to all the staff who are involved in handoffs and will, through direct observation and interviews, determine that this is actually being done consistently.

On September 12, 2017, the Joint Commission issued "Sentinel Event Alert 58: Inadequate Handoff Communication."[3] The alert was an acknowledgment that failed handoffs continued to be a long-standing problem in health care. The Joint Commission's sentinel event database includes reports of inadequate handoff communication causing adverse events, including wrong-site surgery, delay in treatment, falls, and medication errors.

The alert stated that handoffs should be conducted in a high-quality manner for every patient, every day, with every transition of care. It included "8 Tips for High-Quality Hand-Offs," one of which was to conduct handoffs face-to-face in a designated location, a "zone of silence," free from interruptions. The alert also focused on organizational culture and the role of leadership. It noted that it is incumbent that leadership demonstrate a commitment to successful handoffs and make successful handoffs an organizational priority and expectation.

There is an elaborate protective sheath over hospital patients woven of handoffs, taking time-outs in surgery—before the induction of anesthesia, before the first cut, and before they leave the operating room; asking patients for their name and date of birth before giving a medication, then scanning both the ID bracelet and the medication. We cosign heparin drip changes, the amount of insulin we're giving. When we give blood, we read aloud to each other the patient's name, the unit number, donor and patient blood type, date of expiration. The CNO and the house supervisor breached that sheath.

It was a sentinel event because the patient's death was not related to the natural course of her illness or underlying condition. Since 1997, the Joint Commission has mandated a root cause analysis (RCA) for all sentinel events.

RCA is credited to the founder of Toyota, Sakichi Toyoda, who was called the "Japanese Thomas Edison." The technique Toyoda developed was called the Five Whys. You ask "why" five times until the main cause of the problem is revealed. The Five Whys method developed by Toyoda was first used during the development of Toyota's manufacturing processes in 1958. Toyota required all new employees to learn about this process as part of their initiation into the Toyota Production System.[4]

The RCA was held in Auditorium A on the first floor. It's a large room with big windows facing south to Montgomery. There were several long tables arranged in a rectangle. There were about 30 people seated at the tables. The C-team, nurse managers, people from HR, quality, risk management, ER nurses. Maybe legal people. No physicians. I sat near the CNO and the house supervisor. The director of quality began the meeting. She reconstructed the event: the time in the ER; how the patient deteriorated, became hypotensive; how, because she was so sick, she needed two nurses to take care of her, which was causing problems treating other patients; the transport to the ICU; the code and her eventual death.

The emergency department educator spoke next. She talked about how busy the ER was. It was full. She said she had a nursing student with her that day and the ER nurses taking care of the patient thought it would be a good learning experience for the student so they gave her report and left. She said the CNO and the house supervisor were in the ER. They saw that the patient had ICU orders. They decided to transport the patient to the ICU themselves.

When she finished, there was quiet. The CNO didn't speak. Quality didn't say anything. I introduced myself as the patient's ICU nurse that day. I said that hospital protocol calls for a bedside handoff from the ER nurse to the ICU nurse. I said that in other hospitals where I've worked, when an ER patient is waiting to go to the ICU and the ER is busy, we would send a nurse to get report and transfer the patient ourselves. I then said the Levophed wasn't infusing and the pump was on pause.

A C-team member spoke next. She didn't respond to what I said. She started talking about the policy of decompressing the ER, when it began, the criteria for it. Then about other policies to deal with overcrowding in the ER like triaging, fast tracking, and cohorting. She talked about the ER policy of reacting to a surge, how the policy was developed, who could authorize it. How surge levels are based on the National Emergency Department Overcrowding Scale score. That surge codes are communicated by hospital-wide email and overhead page.

Misdirection is the secret of all magic acts. Misdirection is a form of deception where the performer draws audience attention to one thing to distract it from another. The British magician Nevil Maskelyne said, "It consists admittedly in misleading the spectator's senses, in order to screen from detection certain details for which secrecy is required." In *The Encyclopedia of Magic and Magicians*, author T. A. Waters writes that misdirection uses the limits of the human mind to give the wrong picture and memory.[5]

They weren't going to talk about why the CNO and the house supervisor precipitously and irresponsibly transported the patient, the breach of continuity of care, the breaking of the protocol of handoff, why the Levophed wasn't running. They were going to talk about processes, policies. They knew why she died. They called me and I told them. They called to figure out how to keep it a secret. RCA is designed to answer three questions: What happened? Why did it happen? What can be done to prevent it from happening again? The product of the RCA is an action plan that identifies the strategies that the hospital intends to implement in order to reduce the risk of a similar event occurring in the future. The RCA ended without saying why it happened. No plan came out of it.

RCA shares the principle of just culture in focusing primarily on systems and processes, not on individual behavior. The objective of an RCA is not to assign individual blame. But just cultures have zero tolerance for reckless behavior. What the CNO and the house supervisor did, transporting a critically ill patient on a Levophed drip, without a clinical nurse, without a respiratory therapist, was reckless.

A few months later, a postpartum patient was transferred from Labor and Delivery to the ICU with neurological changes. They did an MRI. It was suspicious for a stroke. The hospitalist arranged to transfer her to the neurology service at Lovelace Medical Center. They had an accepting physician and an assigned room and were about to arrange for ambulance transport when the CNO came into the unit and stopped the transfer. There was a lot of activity and discussion outside her room. The hospitalist, the CNO, the nurse. I went into her room because her pump was beeping. Her mother was trying to talk to her. She wasn't responding. Her head was drooping like sunflowers in heat. Her eyes were closed. Her Foley bag was hanging from the bed frame. It was bulging with urine clear as water. Central diabetes insipidus is a lack of the antidiuretic hormone ADH. It leads to excessive production of very dilute urine. It has several causes, including a brain tumor or an ischemic stroke. It can cause a life-threatening loss of body fluids and electrolytes.

Then I remembered an incident several months before that at the time made no impression on me. I had a patient with expressive aphasia who was diagnosed with a stroke by MRI. We were preparing to transfer her to the University of New Mexico Hospital.

We were waiting for a bed. I was charting at my computer when the CNO suddenly appeared in front of it. I remember her smiling and saying, "We can't keep her?" I thought she was kidding and I said, "No. We don't have neurology."

I wondered now why the CNO was suddenly in the ER and the ICU, involved in patient care, in clinical decision-making. Transporting a critically ill patient. Stopping a transfer. Trying to keep a patient we didn't have the ability to care for.

Eileen Appelbaum and Rosemary Batt call it alignment.[6]

The goal of the private equity firm is to maximize financial returns to the shareholders. To achieve this goal, the general partners want to align the interests of the managers of the company with those of the firm and its investors. It's called governance engineering. The term refers to changes the private equity firm makes to the compensation package and benefits of the management team of the portfolio company to align their incentives with those of the private equity owners.

To make managers think and act like owners, the private equity firm turns them into owners.[7] Private equity companies introduce performance-based compensation and bonuses that reward executives and managers for hitting their financial targets. The private equity firm also gives managers generous stock options, which provide the managers an equity stake in the company. Equity stake means ownership. Stock options realign the interests and identities of managers. They shift managers' allegiance from the corporation's purpose and stability to a commitment to maximize shareholder value and their personal wealth as shareholders. Their identities as organizational professionals are supplanted by their self-interest and identities as individual shareholders.[8] These incentives "may detach the senior team from employees, managers and other groups with whom they had implicit contracts and relationships based on trust."[9] The portfolio company's managers essentially become the private equity owners' "agents," their decisions and activity closely monitored by the fund's general partners. The promise to these senior managers is significant wealth if they can meet the private equity owners' performance targets. If they fail to do so, they will be terminated.

The following passage is from Ardent's prospectus, under the section "Our Competitive Strengths":

> Experienced and Aligned Management Team Supported by Strong Equity Sponsorship. Our management team averages over 25 years of healthcare industry experience, with significant experience in managing, acquiring and integrating hospitals. Our management team has consistently demonstrated an ability to improve the operating performance and competitive position of our hospitals. Additionally, our management team owns a significant equity interest in the Company, further aligning their interests in future growth.[10]

This passage is from the "Our Operations and Services" section:

> Our senior management team has extensive experience in operating multi-facility hospital networks and focuses on strategic planning for our facilities. We group our hospitals into divisions with focused local management teams that provide guidance and oversight. Each of our hospitals' local management teams are generally comprised of a chief executive officer, chief financial officer and chief nursing officer or director of nursing. Local management teams, in consultation with our corporate staff, develop annual operating plans setting forth revenue growth strategies through the expansion of offered services, as well as plans to improve operating efficiencies and reduce costs. We believe that the ability of the local management team to identify and meet the needs of our patients, medical staff and the community as a whole is critical to the success of our hospitals. We base the compensation for each local management

team in part on its ability to achieve the clinical quality and financial goals set forth in the annual operating plan. . . .

We provide our local management with corporate assistance in maintaining systematic policies and procedures at each hospital we acquire in order to improve clinical and financial performance. These policies include ethics, quality assurance, safety and compliance programs, supply and equipment purchasing and leasing contracts, managed care contracting, accounting, financial and clinical systems, governmental reimbursement, personnel management, resource management and employee benefits. These uniform policies and procedures are designed to provide us with consistent management and financial reports for all our facilities and facilitate the performance evaluation of each facility.[11]

Appelbaum and Batt write about the control function of debt, how it curbs "managerial opportunism."[12] By that they mean the need to service debt constrains the impulse of managers to invest earnings into the company in terms of wages, benefits, workforce development, and new technology. Debt is a force acting on corporate executives, CNOs, and CEOs to cut costs, generate revenue, and increase cash flow, making them act like the owners private equity wants them to be. If the RCA had been done in the original Toyota way, the Five Whys, it would have revealed why the CNO and the house supervisor were in the ER, why they took it upon themselves to transfer a critically ill patient—a decision that led to her death—and why they violated the hospital's protocol designed to ensure patient safety. They weren't thinking of the patient's welfare; they were thinking of the financial consequences of the patient continuing to be in the ER.

The American College of Emergency Physicians defines a "boarded patient" as "a patient who remains in the emergency department after the patient has been admitted or placed into observation status at the facility, but has not been transferred to an inpatient or observation unit."[13] Boarding is the primary cause of overcrowding. It also has financial consequences. A study in the *Annals of Emergency Medicine* found that "a 1-hour reduction in ED boarding time would result in $9,693 to $13,298 of additional daily revenue from capturing left without being seen and diverted ambulance patients."[14]

Mark Reiter is residency program director of emergency medicine for the University of Tennessee and past president of the American Academy of Emergency Medicine, an advocacy group for practitioners. "Private equity-backed health care has been a disaster for patients and for doctors," he told NBC News. "Many decisions are made for what is going to maximize profits for the private equity company, rather than what is best for the patient, what is best for the community."[15]

11

One Coyote

Her name was Regina Montoya. I never took care of her, but I saw her every day. You couldn't help it. She was in 228 right across from where the hospitalists sit in the middle of the unit. Two twenty-nine and 228 are the smallest rooms. Her bed was less than five feet from the glass doors. You could see the expression on her face. If her eyes were open or closed. How fast she was breathing. At first, if you asked about her, someone would just say "heroin." Not even "OD" or "withdrawal." Just "heroin." Then the story was that she was trying to withdraw at home and her friend was giving her Neurontin in Gatorade.

Some days, over half the unit is substance abuse. It's like there was a leak in a pipe in your basement and now the basement is flooded and water is rising into your kitchen. The alcoholics are either withdrawing or bleeding. Every time they come in, it's like the next chapter in the book of their disease. It starts out with abdominal pain. Hepatomegaly is an enlarged liver. Then they're found down somewhere. Withdraw. Go into delirium tremens. We get their ammonia down with lactulose. The next chapter is gastrointestinal bleed. We scope them. Band their varices. Keep them one more day to see if they rebleed. Then cirrhosis, ascites. And then the end.

Sometimes one of the squares on the whiteboard will say CIWA, which stands for Clinical Institute Withdrawal Assessment for Alcohol. It's an evaluation tool to assess the severity of withdrawal. It consists of 10 questions. You ask the patient if they know where they are; the date; if they're nauseous, having tremors, anxiety; if they have tactile disturbances like itching, pins-and-needles sensations; if they're hearing sounds they know are not there. A score more than 8 and you can give them Ativan. The higher the score, the more Ativan. Sometimes we see where it's headed and you need to cut it off before they go into full-blown delirium tremens, so we give them what we think will work and make a score that fits. When you ask them how much they drink, they'll say, "I quit." You ask them when and they say, "Yesterday." If they do say how much they drink, we triple it.

And then there's drugs. Every few years, like a new car model, there's a different one. Heroin and crack are used cars. Meth is a Honda CR-V. Reliable. A steady seller. Fentanyl is a Prius. The next generation. They come in with abscesses, bodies tattooed with blotches from skin popping, rotten and missing teeth of meth mouth. They're part of the landscape of Albuquerque. You see them walking shirtless down Central, prostrate at a bus stop on Menaul. It used to be if you did heroin or meth, you were an outlaw, but now they work, have jobs. I had a patient who installed solar panels. I heard him on the phone to his boss. "I'll be back soon, better than ever." Another said she was a waitress at El Pinto on Rio Grande. One a teller at Wells Fargo. They're parents with kids. They deliver the mail.

Morning in the unit. Shift change. Nurses huddle in twos giving report. Lydia the housekeeper is pushing her cart to clean 225. I can see into 228. She's sitting up, hunched, desperate breathing. Air hunger. Oxygen-starved lungs sucking down the skin by her clavicle like a winch. Eyes staring wild with fear. She's on an Oxy-Mask. It usually goes nasal cannula, face mask, airvo, OxyMask, BiPaP (bilevel positive airway pressure), then the ventilator. It's a descent. Something happened during the night. Maybe she aspirated, had a pulmonary embolism. She needs to be intubated. They're waiting. Sanchez is the pulmonologist today. He's sitting at a computer talking to the pharmacist. The respiratory therapist is at the door with the ventilator. Gavin has her today. Sanchez tells Gavin the drugs he wants. He gets the rapid sequence intubation kit from the Pyxis. The kit has drugs. It has Versed for sedation, succinylcholine to paralyze. Fentanyl for pain. Then some syringes, needles, and saline flushes. Gavin draws the drugs up into syringes, then tapes each vial to its syringe to keep track of what's what. He opens the saline flushes' plastic wrappers so he's ready. American bull riding has been called the most dangerous 8 seconds in sports. Intubation is the most dangerous 60 seconds in medicine. You're holding them over an abyss. They're paralyzed. Can't breathe on their own. Sometimes it goes into their stomach and you need to pull it back. Oxygen saturation levels dropping 68 . . . 60.

They put a pillow under her shoulder to hyperextend the neck. With his left hand, Sanchez puts a curved metal blade with a light on the tip into her mouth to move the tongue out of the way and light up the airway. In his right hand, like a stiletto, he holds a plastic tube with a metal stylet inside. He's looking for the cords. He'll thread the tube through them into her trachea. He's skilled. He's in. He pulls the stylet out. The respiratory therapist bags her. With his stethoscope, Gavin listens to her stomach first and then her lungs. He nods and says, "Bilateral sounds." They connect her to the ventilator. She's still. Her breathing steadies. It's a kind of peace.

Days go by. She has a large family. Nice people. One day the mother brings in food for the unit: a huge bowl of chicken salad. Another bowl of fruit salad. Bags of Lay's potato chips. Rolls. Enough to feed the whole unit, both shifts, for more than a day.

Another day. They're doing an EEG in the room. I asked her nurse why. She said she was unresponsive. Stiff neck. I ask the physician if she has meningitis. He shrugs his shoulders and says she's already on antibiotics. They do a CT. It shows multiple cerebellar infarcts. A cerebral infarction is a stroke where something blocks the flow of blood and brain cells die from a lack of oxygen. "Probably septic emboli. A septic shower," Gavin says. Staphylococcus bacteria live on your skin and on mucous membranes like the one inside your nose. They're harmless there. But if they get into your body, into your bloodstream, they can cause life-threatening infection, inflammation, death. Staph bacteria enter the blood of IV drug users through the broken skin from needle punctures. They can travel to the heart and cause endocarditis, inflammation of the valves and the inner lining of the heart. They form grape-like clusters. The word "staph" is from ancient Greek, *staphyle*, "bunch of grapes." Small clumps break off. They travel through the bloodstream to the kidneys, lungs, and brain, where they block blood flow. I ask Gavin why she's not going to the University of New Mexico Hospital (UNM). "They say there's nothing they can do for her," he says.

"She should be at UNM."

"You're preaching to the choir. Every day in rounds I bring it up."

There would be a threshold or a boundary we would reach with a patient when we knew not just that the patient needed an intervention we couldn't provide but that we had reached the limit of our care, our imaginings, and the patient needed to be at UNM, where they had not just new but better eyes and minds. It was tacitly understood in morning rounds by everyone: the nurse, the physician, case management. The physician would order the transfer. We would call the house supervisor to let her know. Administration would sign off. The house supervisor would call the transfer hospital, which would give us a room, tell us the receiving physician, the name of the nurse, a number to call report. Then we would call the ambulance. It was automatic. Then it stopped being automatic.

Paul Starr's Pulitzer Prize–winning *The Social Transformation of American Medicine* traces the rise of medicine as a sovereign profession. It's an epic of progress, but it is also a tale of how the medical profession was able to maintain its autonomy against the threat of corporate and bureaucratic interference. Physicians "opposed corporate enterprise in medical practice not only because they wanted to preserve their autonomy, but also because they wanted to prevent the emergence of any intermediary or third party that might keep for itself the profits potentially available in the practice of medicine."[1] The medical profession was successful in influencing the development of hospitals, health insurance, and health maintenance organizations so that they did not impinge on its professional autonomy. It was aided by the "corporate practice of medicine" doctrine, developed at the state level, which prohibited or restricted the ownership of medical practice by anyone nonlicensed. The intent was to prevent corporate ownership of medical practices and to promote the physician-patient relationship. Between 1915 and 1917, several states passed laws that prohibited corporations from engaging in the commercial practice of medicine, even if they employed licensed physicians, "on the grounds that a corporation could not be licensed to practice and that commercialism in medicine violated 'sound public policy.'"[2] For years the medical profession was able to secure its autonomy. Starr describes these years as "escape from the corporation."[3]

The Social Transformation of American Medicine was written in 1982. The final section of the book is titled "The Coming of the Corporation." Starr saw the beginnings of an erosion of medical sovereignty and the early stages of a corporate transformation of American medicine. Corporations were beginning to consolidate what had been a decentralized hospital system. Traditional independent general hospitals, governed by their own board of directors, administrators, and medical staff, were disappearing, being absorbed by large multihospital systems in what would become an industry dominated by huge health-care conglomerates.

The rise of a corporate ethos in medical care will have a profound impact on the practice of medicine as well as "on the culture of medical care institutions" such as the hospital.[4] Physicians will lose much of the autonomy the profession had so assiduously protected. There will be more scrutiny and regulation of work in terms of revenue generated or patients seen per hour; physicians will be evaluated for their productivity; mistakes will be less tolerated because of corporate liability for malpractice. Corporate management will explore techniques for changing the behavior of physicians, getting them to accept management's expectations and values and integrate them into their everyday work. Starr saw the method as subliminal, not overt: "That way they do not need to be supervised and do not sense any loss of control."[5] Just as sociologists have studied the "professional socialization" that takes place in medical school as students internalize the values and attitudes of experienced physicians, they would in the future study "corporate socialization" as physicians introject the way corporate management wants things done. As Starr observes, "Another key issue will be the boundary between medical and business decisions; when both medical and economic decisions are relevant, which will prevail and who will decide? Much will depend on the external forces driving the organization."[6]

Starr saw this as the future toward which American medicine was headed.

That future has come to pass. Private equity is the contemporary form of the corporate future augured in Starr's book. At Lovelace Women's Hospital, corporate socialization began at the executive level and gradually extended to the practice of medicine. Laura Katz Olson writes about how "the doctor-patient relationship is increasingly sculpted to PE's [private equity's] extreme economic orthodoxy."[7] Private equity's emphasis on generating revenue rather than doing what is best for the patient affected the decision not to transfer a critically ill patient to a higher level of care.

The following is from Ardent's prospectus: "In pursuing our business and financial objectives, we pay close attention to a number of performance measures and operational factors. Hospital revenues depend primarily upon inpatient occupancy levels, the ancillary services and therapy programs ordered by physicians and provided to patients, the volume of outpatient procedures and the charges and negotiated payment rates for such services."[8]

Any patient transferred from a hospital is lost revenue, but a ventilated patient is a significant loss. From a financial standpoint, a ventilated patient is lucrative. Ventilated patients have a substantially higher cost and greater length of stay than nonventilated patients. The mean length of stay of a ventilated patient is between 14 and 16 days; the mean hospital costs are between $34,000 and $40,559.

One day she's incontinent of stool. It's liquid. Gavin asks me to help clean her up. "Broke her leg," he says. "Tib-fib." He pulls down the sheet to show me the scar just below her knee. "She's flaccid on the right." I open her eyelids. Her eyes deviate up and toward the left. "She's looking at the lesion. Are they going to scan her?" We turn her on her side and I hold her. Even though she's sedated, he talks to her, tells her what he's going to do, every step. "I'm going to turn you on your side. I'm going to wipe you with a wet washcloth."

They do an MRI. I bring it up on the computer. The brain is divided into the left and right cerebral hemispheres. There's a cloud of dead tissue in the left hemisphere. In a stroke, the eyes deviate. It's called the Prévost sign. The symptom was described by Swiss neurologist Jean-Louis Prévost in 1868. It tells you where the stroke is. Patients with hemisphere lesions look toward their lesion. Patients with an injury to the thalamus look away from their lesions.

It's seven thirty in the morning two days later. Gavin tells me
her pupils aren't reacting and asks if I could assess her. The ventilator is set to deliver so many breaths a minute, 12 to 16. They're
called machine breaths. But you can breathe spontaneously on
your own as well. They're called patient breaths. She has no patient breaths. I lift her eyelids. I shine the light from my iPhone
onto them. Her pupils are 4 mm. They don't react. I touch the tip
of a two-by-two gauze to the edge of her cornea. It should make
her eyelid twitch. It's called the blink reflex. It doesn't. The ventilator has a closed suction system. It's called Ballard suction. It's
a catheter that's protected inside a sterile sleeve. I pass the suction catheter the length of the endotracheal tube to the carina.
It should make her cough. Nothing. Then I test for doll's eyes.

If you turn a doll's head side to side, the eyes move in the opposite direction of the head movement. It's called the oculoce-
phalic reflex. It's a reflex eye movement that stabilizes images on
the retina during head movement so the image stays on the center of the visual field. When the head moves to the right, the eyes
move to the left, and vice versa, so they are always looking forward. A loss of this reflex means the eyes stay fixed and turn with
the head and don't move back to the midline. Having doll's eyes
is a good thing. Not having doll's eyes indicates severe brainstem
injury. I lift her eyelids with the thumb and index finger of my right
hand and turn her head quickly to the right. Her eyes remain stationary. To the left. Stationary.

Pupils fixed. No cough. Negative doll's eyes. I say to Gavin,
"She's dead."

I look into the unit. The nurse who had her last night is still here.
Rachel. She's talking to another nurse, who's seated at her computer. They're laughing about something.

I go with Gavin to CT. Sarah is bagging her. Back in the unit
Gavin says, "I wish I had seen it yesterday." I know what he means.
That there are signs. When I was travel nursing, I did some shifts

in the Neuroscience ICU at the University of California San Francisco. One day a nurse's patient's pupil blew. Went to the operating room right away. I complimented her. "It's great to catch it when it happens." She smiled and said, "It's best to see it before it happens."

I open the patient's chart. Every two hours, the night nurse charted her pupils 2 mm and reactive. She didn't die at seven o'clock this morning. The radiology doc calls to say the CT is bad. Massive cerebral bleed. Medically, it's called hemorrhagic transformation of embolic lesions.

The hospitalist is Dr. Anderson. He's calling the Physician Access Line Service (PALS) at UNM. It was created so community physicians could consult with UNM physicians and get help with a diagnosis or treatment or arrange a transfer. PALS is available 24/7. He doesn't know what to do. I sit close to hear the conversation. He's telling PALS the history, the MRI, the CT scan this morning. Then he listens for several minutes. He puts the phone down.

"We need the brain death form. We need to follow the algorithm. Do the tests."

I ask Maria to call Lovelace Medical Center and fax it to us.

Death has changed. Death was once when your heart stopped. It was called "heart-lung" death. Then it was "whole brain death": irreversible cessation of functioning of the entire brain. Death had slipped its moorings. Death was different state by state, like the drinking age or sales tax. You could be an intensive care patient being transferred from a hospital in Newark to one in Boston and be alive in New Jersey, dead in Connecticut, and alive again in Massachusetts. There were commissions and studies. In 1976, the Harvard Ad Hoc Committee on Irreversible Coma. In 1981, the President's Commission study *Defining Death: A Report on the Medical, Legal and Ethical Issues in the Determination of Death*. Also in 1981, the Uniform Determination of Death Act to help states determine when someone was dead. Encroached upon by advances in medicine, death changed again. Cardiac defibrillation, pioneered by the American cardiologist Paul Zoll, delivered electrical shocks to the chest and stopped life-threatening arrhythmias. CPR combined mouth-to-mouth ventilation with chest compressions to maintain blood flow and oxygenation in people with no respirations or heartbeat. The immunosuppressant cyclosporine transformed the nascent science of organ transplantation from research surgery to life-saving treatment. The survival of patients on life support increased the demand and urgency for organ transplantation.

In 1995 the Royal College of Physicians in the United Kingdom suggested a new definition of death based on the irreversible loss of brainstem function alone. Other countries adopted it. Australia, New Zealand, then Brazil. In 2020, an international panel of experts, the World Brain Death Project, published recommendations for the determination of brain death by neurologic criteria. Death became brainstem death.

The brainstem is near the bottom of the brain, at the back of the skull. It looks like a flower stalk. It connects the cerebrum and cerebellum to the spinal cord. It regulates essential life functions such as breathing, heart rate, and blood pressure. It contains 10 of the 12 cranial nerves that start in the brain that control balance, hearing, swallowing, facial movements, fine touch, and taste. If the brainstem doesn't function, consciousness and the ability to breathe are lost. You can be in the ICU, on a ventilator, your heart beating, warm, getting fluid, peeing, and be dead.

The form is eight pages long. Anderson repeats what Gavin and I did. Pupils, cough, doll's eyes. Then the oculovestibular reflex. It's also called the cold caloric test. As for doll's eyes, you stimulate eye movement to see if the reflex that stabilizes the visual field and retinal image is intact. We do it when doll's eyes are negative because it's a stronger stimulus. You do it by injecting ice-cold water into the ear. If the reflex is intact, the eyes will move rapidly away from the stimulated ear and then slowly back. I put a chux and an emesis basin below her left ear. Anderson fills a Toomey syringe with 45 ccs of water from an emesis basin. "Someone needs to hold her eyes open," he says. Gavin lifts her lids with his thumb and index fingers. Opening her eyes makes her look startled. Alive. Like someone just told her something she couldn't believe—her best friend told her she was pregnant; her boyfriend told her he was taking her to Naples—and she gasps, her eyes go wide. Anderson injects the water into her ear. There are small chunks of ice in the syringe. You almost expect her eyes to move. They don't. You have to wait five minutes for the oculovestibular system to re-equilibrate before doing the other ear. They don't move.

The apnea test is the last and most important test because it's not about whether your pupils react, if you blink, or if you cough; it's whether you can breathe. Apnea is the absence of breathing. The stimulation to breathe is triggered not by low oxygen but by the need to get rid of carbon dioxide. Normal carbon dioxide levels in the blood are 35 to 45 mm HG. In apnea testing, we let the carbon dioxide rise to greater than 60. No spontaneous respiratory effort with a partial pressure of carbon dioxide greater than 60 is apnea and the diagnosis of brainstem death. First we hyper-oxygenate her with 100% oxygen for 10 minutes. Gavin draws blood for the arterial blood gas analysis. He feels for the pulse of the artery with his index finger, then aims the needle at a 45-degree angle just below where he feels it. Bright red blood spurts into the syringe. Sarah runs the blood in the room on her machine. The patient's carbon dioxide level is 40. Normal. I cut the end of the oxygen tubing where the nasal prongs are. Sarah disconnects the ventilator. I thread it down to the end of the tube to the carina and run the oxygen flow meter at 10 liters a minute. At five minutes, Gavin draws blood for an arterial blood gas analysis. Her partial pressure of carbon dioxide is 62. At ten minutes, he draws

another. The partial pressure of carbon dioxide is 74. Sarah re-
connects the ventilator. She never takes a breath.

I see Anderson talking to the family. I ask Gavin what they're
going to do.

"Withdraw. They're waiting for a brother."

"What did the mother say when he told her?"

"She understood. She said she was a very active person, always
doing something, and she wouldn't have wanted not to be like
that."

The brother is in Taos. It's almost three hours away. Maria had
called for a bereavement cart. A thermos of coffee. A pitcher of
water. Bags of chips. Cookies. Fruit. Kristen brings extra chairs
into the room. I help Gavin clean her up. We have the family wait
just outside the room. Wash her face. Comb her hair. Change her
gown. The last image. The family's back.

"Can you put her scapular back?" her mother asks.

It's on a side table. I lay it on her chest.

"Not like that." She gives me kind smile. "It goes around her
neck."

It's a leather cord with two leather-framed images the size of a
postage stamp. She can tell I don't know what it is.

"That's Jesus and the Virgin Mary. You go right to heaven."

For the next few hours friends come, from their lives, from jobs,
homes, as if in response to the Islamic call to prayer that goes out
from the mosque. Two women. A couple. One man alone walking
slowly, his head down. They move among us all morning, a quiet
stream of grief flowing in and out of the unit until by early afternoon everyone had seen her and the stream of grief disappeared
and there was only family. Mother, sister, son, daughter, aunts and
uncles, cousins. A boy in a wheelchair. He's been here before. A
man with him. But he doesn't go into the room. His legs are concentration camp thin. Cerebral palsy. He cries, then stops. Cries,
stops. The man is kneeling next to him. His arm is around the

boy's shoulder. The man's right hand is in a fist and he's gently bouncing it off the boy's knee. But it's a kind gesture, like telling the boy he's strong. The sister kneels and hugs him. He never looks in the room.

The sister is at her side. I see her bend down and kiss her forehead and then lay her head next to her on the pillow. The mother is against the wall at the end of the bed under the clock. Her face is anguished. She has a hospital washcloth in her hands. She raises it to wipe her tears, and when she lowers the cloth it's the same anguished face. Several men are outside. They're standing a little apart from each other. Like they've found the space they needed. They're quietly crying. They seem like those granite boulders near waterfalls that glisten with moisture like they're weeping. You can feel their sadness. What she meant to them. Like they're beads and she was the thread that ran through all of them.

Most people don't die like her. You withdraw. It takes time. They breathe for a while. Only her heart is beating. In the wilderness of her body, only the sound of one coyote. Everywhere else silence. She has a young heart. It beats for a while. They're quiet in the room. The sister is holding her hand. The mother now in a chair next to her. Finally her young heart slows down and stops.

Gavin has to call Donor Services and the Office of Medical Investigation. They sign off. I get busy with an admission. Everyone is gone except the sister. I see a guy with a suit pushing a stretcher come into the unit with the house supervisor and security. The funeral home. Later the room is cleaned, empty, the bed made. They trusted us. They brought us food. When they learned she was dead they didn't get angry. She should have been transferred a week ago. The standard of care for patients with cerebellar infarction is monitoring in a dedicated neuroscience ICU. "These patients need close neurological monitoring and may require neurosurgical intervention."[9] Cerebellar infarction complications include increased intracranial pressure and bleeding of the brain tissue. Cerebellar infarction can cause life-threatening cerebral edema, which produces pressure that can force brain tissue downward into the foramen magnum, the opening in the base of the skull that connects the spinal cord to the brain. It's called brain herniation.

On a CT scan, cerebellar infarction shows up as darker than surrounding tissues. Blood on a CT scan is bright white. Hemorrhagic transformation is diagnosed when areas of cerebellar infarction now appear as cerebellar hemorrhage on CT imaging. Hemorrhagic transformation can occur as a natural progression inasmuch as infarcted cerebral tissue, as in other organs, tends to bleed. It can occur when there is reperfusion of the infarcted area and damaged blood vessels rupture. Or when the blood-brain barrier, a semipermeable membrane that keeps harmful substances from reaching the brain, is disrupted and blood extravasates across it.

In both cases, "timely escalation of treatment is crucial and should be guided by clinical and neuroradiological rationales."[10] The treatment for increased intracranial pressure can escalate from medical management with an osmotic diuretic such as mannitol to reduce cerebral edema, to a ventriculostomy where a catheter is inserted into one of the brain's ventricles to monitor intracranial pressure and drain cerebrospinal fluid, to surgical intervention. "Emergent decompressive surgery by suboccipital craniectomy, with or without partial removal of infarcted tissue, can be life saving and can preserve quality of life."[11]

The treatment of hemorrhagic transformation includes managing blood pressure; controlling bleeding with cryoprecipitate, a plasma derivative rich in clotting factors; and using neurosurgical interventions such as drilling burr holes into the skull and draining blood from the brain through flexible rubber tubes or conducting a hemicraniectomy, in which a large flap of the skull is removed to relieve pressure and evacuate clotted blood.

They told Gavin they weren't going to transfer her because there was nothing they could do for her at UNM. These are the things they could have done for her at UNM. That could have saved her life. All it would have taken was a doctor-to-doctor phone call, an acceptance, a bed, an ambulance ride. They didn't give her that chance.

Ardent has a 69-page Code of Conduct. It begins with a message from the president and CEO, Martin J. Bonick, who says that Ardent culture has always emphasized "doing the right thing." The code includes Ardent's purpose and mission. The purpose: "Caring for people: our patients, their families and one another." The mission: "Ardent Health Services is a premier provider of healthcare services, delivered with *compassion* for patients and their families, with *respect* for employees, physicians and other health professionals, with *accountability* for our fiscal and ethical performance, and with *responsibility* to the communities we serve."[12]

The sections are about "caring," as in "We Care about Each Other," "We Care about Our Industry." One section is "We Care about Our Patients." It has a subsection, "How We Care," which says, "We only transfer a patient if our facility does not have the capacity or capability of treating the patient, or if the patient or guardian requests the transfer. In these cases, the patient is transferred to an appropriate facility after the facility receiving the patient provides formal acceptance."[13]

That sounds good, right? It's what you would expect of an 8-bed ICU in a community hospital where two miles away is a university teaching hospital with three ICUs that have over 20 beds each and resident physicians in every specialty. It's a noble mission. It's one we embraced. We understood who we were as a hospital and what our responsibility was to patients who needed a level of care we couldn't provide.

It was true for many years, but in the years after Ventas bought Ardent, it stopped being true.

12

The Tribe

Her name was Amber Begay. She was a 30-year-old Navajo woman from Gallup admitted for alcohol withdrawal and bilateral knee injuries from falls while intoxicated. Gallup is sometimes called the Indian Capital of the World. It's in the heart of Indian land—Hopi, Zuni, but mostly Navajo. Navajo Nation is the largest federally recognized tribe in the United States. Its 25,000 square miles cover parts of Arizona, New Mexico, and Utah. It's bigger than 10 states. It is estimated that 80% of the adult population has an alcohol problem. Navajo Nation has a no-drinking, no-possession, no-sales ban. Many Navajo will drive off the reservation to bars and liquor stores in Shiprock, Farmington, and Gallup and binge drink. Along the 72 miles of highway between Tuba City, on the Navajo reservation, and Flagstaff to the south, are 149 white crosses that mark the sites of fatal accidents, most caused by alcohol and most of the victims Native Americans.

Food deserts are geographic areas where people don't have access to healthy foods like fresh fruits and vegetables because there are no grocery stores. Then there are medical deserts that lack certain specialties like OB-GYN or cardiology, requiring patients to travel hundreds of miles for care. Gallup is a medical desert. It has no gastroenterologists and few detoxification centers, so the GI bleeders and alcohol withdrawals come to Albuquerque. Because the University of New Mexico Hospital and Presbyterian keep beds open for traumas and high-acuity patients, a lot of them come to us.

Her family is a boyfriend, a mother, two aunts. She has two children back in Gallup. A little tribe. They come and go. Quietly. Carrying blankets. Stay deep into the evening like making a camp at night under the moon.

I helped Gavin turn her once. She was tall, maybe 5'10". Awake. Quiet. I could see the bruises on her knees. Her withdrawal got worse. They put her on the Clinical Institute Withdrawal Assessment for Alcohol protocol. She maybe aspirated and developed respiratory distress. She went from nasal cannula to a regular face mask to an OxyMask. She was constantly pulling the mask off her face, dropping her oxygen level. The nurse who had her said she called the house supervisor and asked for a sitter. She said the supervisor told her, "There's no sitter available. Sitters don't grow on trees."

Sitters are usually the patient care technicians from Med-Surg. We use them for patients who are combative, delirious, confused, suicidal, or withdrawing. Such patients are at risk for getting out of bed and falling; pulling out IVs, Foley catheters, or nasogastric tubes; ripping the EKG electrodes off their chest. They don't use the call bell, so they're incontinent. They're time consuming. You almost can't leave them alone. Sitters keep them in check, keep their oxygen on, don't let them pull lines. Protect them from themselves.

We have another interim ICU manager. One day she was in the unit. She looked into a room where there was a sitter for a patient going through alcohol withdrawal. She scowled and said they were going to get rid of sitters because there's no evidence they prevent falls.

Although data on the patient sitter role is scarce, the significance of the role has steadily increased in health care. Susan B. Frampton is president of the nonprofit organization Planetree, which works with health-care organizations on implementing comprehensive person-centered models of care. According to Frampton, the increased use of patient sitters has been driven by reports published by the Institute of Medicine on quality of care and patient safety and the health-care industry's movement away from punitive measures like restraints and seclusion rooms to deal with combative or at-risk patients. "As our nation tries to do a better job of supporting the needs of behavioral health patients, the role of patient sitters will become even more important than it is currently," says Dr. Frampton. "It will only become more so as the patient-centered movement, which demands hospitals to personalize care, progresses."[1] Sitters should be viewed as important members of the health-care team who are integral to patient safety.

An article on the high rates of bankruptcies among private equity–owned retailers on the online site Retail Dive, "Is the Road to Bankruptcy Paved by Private Equity?," quotes Nick Egelanian, president at SiteWorks: "At the core of these things, they're running an investment firm, not a retail business. The retailer becomes the collateral rather than the actual business you're in."[2]

Ardent is in the investment, not the health-care, business.

Its prospectus is a financial document. There's nothing about disease, illness, pain, suffering, death. Or safety. It's not about the care in health care. About our devotion to patients, the responsibility we feel toward the poor, the vulnerable. It's about investment, revenue. It uses language like "EIDBTA," "Corporate Conversion," "strategic capital investments." It talks about the Anti-Kickback Statute or the Stark Law. It talks about market reach, cost synergies. This is how it talks about patients: "We compute utilization of licensed beds by multiplying admissions by the number of days patients admitted for inpatient treatment stay in our hospitals during the applicable period, then dividing that number by the number of days in such period, and then dividing that number by average licensed beds."[3] It doesn't talk about patient-centered care or about safety. Patient sitters mitigate the fear, anxiety, and terror patients can experience. They prevent falls, injuries, harm. They enhance quality of care. Dr. Frampton notes, "By having these individuals sit with high-needs patients, hospitals can free up some of the time of the highly trained professional staff who are needed to perform other clinical tasks."[4] In the cost-cutting world of private equity, a $12-an-hour sitter is a low-hanging fruit.

With no sitter, the nurse placed bilateral wrist restraints on the patient. They're called soft restraints as opposed to four-point leathers that you lock with a key. They're light blue with a Velcro attachment and two white straps you loop around their wrist, thread through a metal ring, and then tie to the bed frame in a quick-release knot in case they code. They can struggle. They try to lift their arms, arch their backs, thrash their head side to side. Hunch themselves to get their teeth on the straps. You're sedating them with Ativan, Haldol. Maybe Librium as well. You have to monitor them closely. They're at risk for aspirating, asphyxiation, injury. They can stop breathing. We often make them a one-to-one. You have to keep them in sight.

In the 1990s, the use of restraints in the ICU increased in conjunction with the prevalence of more invasive devices such as chest tubes, ventriculostomies, and Swan-Ganz catheters that, if they were to come out, by accident or by a patient removing them, could be life threatening. There's a tipping point in the ICU. Survival is said to be a race between the risks and benefits of life-saving interventions. The saving fluid that floods the lungs. Ventilator-acquired pneumonia. The tipping point for restraints was delirium.

Delirium is a disease of the ICU. It can be caused by sleep deprivation, social isolation, unfamiliar surroundings, the side effects of medications. Symptoms can range from confusion to lethargy to aggression. It can lead to long-term cognitive impairment and death. ICU delirium is associated with increased mortality 0–30 days after hospital discharge.[5] An article in the *Journal of Clinical Nursing* found that restraints, the experience of involuntary immobilization, increased the risk of delirium in the ICU threefold.[6]

Restraints have been exiled to the fringes of medical care. You're supposed to do everything you can to avoid using them. They're intensely scrutinized. Every shift, the house supervisor asks if anybody is in restraints so administration is aware. Quality monitors your charting every day and calls you if you haven't done something. It's one of the first things the Joint Commission survey teams look at. Documentation is exacting. An assessment of the patient every two hours. Justification of their use every four. The order has to be renewed every day. They must be discontinued at the earliest possible time. Both the Centers for Medicare and Medicaid Services and the Joint Commission have adopted patient care standards to minimize restraint use. Restraints are only used as a last resort. The situation has to be life threatening. The threat of patient violence imminent.

Then there's the ethical issue. The Centers for Medicare and Medicaid Services have criteria that hospitals must meet in order to participate in and be reimbursed by Medicare and Medicaid programs. They're called Conditions of Participation, and they are Part 482 of the Code of Federal Regulations (CFR).

Title 42, Section 482.13, of the CFR is titled "Condition of Participation: Patient's Rights." It says a hospital must protect and promote each patient's rights. Some of these rights are the right to privacy, the right to confidentiality, the right to participate in the development and implementation of the plan of care. 42 CFR 482.13 has eight subsections, a–h. Sections e and f are about restraints. They say "all patients have the right to be free from restraint or seclusion, of any form, imposed as a means of coercion, discipline, convenience, or retaliation by staff. Restraint or seclusion may only be imposed to ensure the immediate physical safety of the patient, a staff member, or others." They also state that "the type or technique of restraint or seclusion must be the least restrictive intervention" to protect the patient or staff from harm.[7] The patient has the right to the safe use of restraints and to a staff trained in the application, monitoring, assessment, and care for a patient in restraints.

It's early afternoon. She's in 229 directly across from where the unit secretary sits. The curtain's drawn. Her nurse is sitting at her computer behind the secretary in the nurses' station. The secretary suddenly turns to her and says, "Your patient is in asystole!" She's flatline on the monitor. They find her with the OxyMask off. Not breathing. In cardiac arrest. They call a code. They get her back. Intubate her. Days go by. She never regains consciousness. The family decides to withdraw support. She dies within minutes.

James T. Reason first described the Swiss cheese model to explain system failures in his 1990 book *Human Error*.[8] It likens systems to multiple slices of Swiss cheese stacked side by side, where the risk of an accident becoming a reality is lessened by the series of barriers layered behind one another. The holes represent weaknesses in individual parts of the system. They continually vary in size and position across the slices. If the holes momentarily align, there is a "a trajectory of accident opportunity,"[9] and a hazard can pass through holes in all of the barriers, leading to harm.

The nurse had transferred from Med-Surg three months ago. Because we had lost experienced staff in the ICU, she was oriented by a nurse who wasn't a trained preceptor. Bedside computer charting is the standard of care in the contemporary ICU. It's called point-of-care documentation. Some ICUs have fixed computers in a windowed alcove between two rooms. Some have wall-attached computers in the rooms. We have computers on wheels that enable us to go room to room. Point-of-care documentation means you record information as you obtain it and document care as you provide it while at the patient's bedside. Real-time documentation is essential to detect signs of change and initiate rapid, appropriate interventions. Gavin, Kristen, and I chart in or just outside our patient's room. Point of care. This nurse wasn't trained that way. She sat at her computer in the nurses' station. She practiced like she was still on Med-Surg. Med-Surg monitoring typically consists of intermittent spot checks every 2–3 hours. Face-to-face evaluation is an imperative across the duration of the use of restraints. A patient who is restrained must be seen face-to-face by a physician within 1 hour after the initiation of the restraints to evaluate "the patient's immediate situation, the patient's reaction to the intervention, the patient's medical and behavioral condition, the need to continue or terminate the restraint."[10] After 24 hours, before writing a new order for the use of restraints, a physician must see and assess the patient. Even though her patient was restrained, on a high level of oxygen, and at high risk, the nurse was not charting at point of care, not visually evaluating her.

Every hospital has clinical educators who are devoted to specific areas like the ICU, the emergency department, the NICU. Clinical educators in the hospital have multiple responsibilities. They evaluate educational needs for their clinical areas, ensure competency of staff by skill testing, conduct in-services on new products and devices, ensure standards of care are being maintained. They also monitor the orientation of new nurses. Clinical educators select the preceptor for a new employee, meet weekly with them, evaluate progress, gauge needs, and check off competencies. The educator is like a screen ensuring that someone doesn't get into the ICU who isn't ready. Preceptees are not allowed to be on their own until they've had experience with several drips, know how they're administered, how to titrate them; know the ventilator, the different modes, how to do a spontaneous breathing trial; know that when you're giving blood, you have to stay in the room for the first 15 minutes in case the patient has a hemolytic transfusion reaction. They have to show they've made the transition from Med-Surg monitoring to ICU monitoring, that they understand what's at stake.

One-third of nurses who come to the ICU from Med-Surg don't succeed in making the transition. They usually go back to Med-Surg to get more experience. We had been without an educator for several months. She left for a clinical instructor job at the University of New Mexico Hospital's Valencia campus in Los Lunas and, in a cost-cutting move, the hospital didn't replace her. There was no one to supervise the nurse's orientation, ensure that she was competent, exercised good clinical judgment, followed the protocol for restraints. With no educator, we lost the gatekeeper.

42 CFR Section 482.13(f)(2)(iv), on staff training requirements for a patient in restraints, states the hospital must require staff to have education, training, and demonstrated knowledge in "how to recognize and respond to signs of physical and psychological distress (for example, positional asphyxia)."[11]

No sitter. No educator. Poor training. Private equity decisions lined the holes up.

We have alcoholics who go through severe withdrawal. They go into withdrawal three to seven days after their last drink. They start off slow. Tremors. Hands shaking when they eat. See spiders on their blanket. Their heart rate picks up. Then they're wild. Pulling out IVs. Incontinent. Crawling over the siderails. You're giving Ativan. They can break through and you might be giving 8 or 10 milligrams every 15 minutes two or three times to put them back down. They're on ventilators. Sometimes for weeks. They have Foleys, feeding tubes. You think there's no way they'll be who they were. But they get extubated, go to rehab, and then one day one of the docs will say, "Do you remember so-and-so? He went home yesterday. He's doing great." She was 30. In relatively good health. She had two kids who will never know her. Thirty-year-old alcoholics who go through withdrawal don't die.

Luke Johnson, manager of the private equity firm Risk Capital Partners, wrote in the *Financial Times* that private equity is "a pure capitalist pursuit in which investors buy companies and try to sell them for a capital gain. There is an intense focus on returns for shareholders, enriching management, and less concern for citizens as a whole."[12]

Nursing has a closer relationship with patients and families than medicine. Charles Rosenberg wrote of the early hospital that society reconstructed itself within it: "At least two subcultures coexisted within the hospital: that of the patients and attendants who cared for them, on the one hand, and that of the hospital's lay trustees, medical staff and superintendent." He continued, "The recruitment of hospital physicians . . . guaranteed a maximum social distance between doctor and patient."[13] It's true to this day. We come from the same soil. Their stories, their struggles, their hopes. Their lives echo in ours.

Laudato si' (Praise Be to You) is the second encyclical of Pope Francis.[14] It was published on June 18, 2015. The subtitle of the encyclical is "On Care for Our Common Home." In it, the pope decries the capitalist system that makes goods disposable rather than durable so that consumers must continue to repurchase items. The pope calls it a "throwaway culture." He blames a reckless pursuit of profits for the exploitation and destruction of the environment. In the throwaway culture, it's not only unwanted items but unwanted people who are discarded as waste: the unborn, the elderly, and the poor. Human lives, people on the margins of society, are treated as disposable.

In James Salter's *Light Years*, Viri says to his wife, Nedra, "The best education comes from knowing only one book. Purity comes from that, and proportion, and the comfort of always having an example close at hand."[15] That one book for me would be James Agee's *Let Us Now Praise Famous Men*.

In 1938, Agee was commissioned by *Fortune* magazine to go to Alabama to write about the people who were the poorest of the poor in America: the southern sharecroppers. Agee writes about three families on a hill: the Grudgers, with whom he stays; the Woods, whose daughters are Emma and Annie Mae; and the Ricketts. Agee lives with them less than four weeks, seeing them "intimately and constantly," going to sleep, waking, undressing, eating meals, rolling cigarettes. He finds the world of the sharecroppers more complex than he had anticipated, more dignified. In the preface, Agee writes, the "nominal subject is North American cotton tenantry as examined in the daily living of three representative white tenant families."[16] He struggled to write the book. "Actually, the effort is to recognize the stature of a portion of unimagined existence and to contrive techniques proper to its recording, communication, analysis and defense." Finally Agee concludes, "More essentially, this is an independent inquiry into certain normal predicaments of human divinity."[17] The title is from Ecclesiastes.

Even though they are poor, without any real hope, they don't seem to want for anything; uneducated, they have an innate wisdom; trapped, they are not without pride. Agee begins to see in their lives dignity and beauty. He sees them as noble human beings, folk heroes, "famous men." The photographer Walker Evans, whose 37 black-and-white photographs introduce the book, said of Agee, "After a while, in a round-about way, you discovered that, to him, human beings were at least possibly immortal and literally sacred souls."[18]

You see the homeless all over Albuquerque. On Lomas pushing shopping carts piled high with everything they own. Sleeping under the Siberian elms in Bataan Park. On medians flying a sign. That's what they call it. A piece of cardboard. "Looking for a warm room tonight." "A little means a lot. God Bless." Haikus of suffering. Some of them wave. Some walk the line of waiting cars at a red light. I keep fives in the ashtray.

We always have a small group of them. Right now it's Laura Castilla, Anthony King, and Carlos Vigil. If you need to start an IV, they'll tell you what vein to use and where not to go. They come in every month or two, and then they don't come in anymore because they're dead. They're savvy. They work you, but I don't mind. They'll tell you morphine doesn't work and they need Dilaudid. It's as needed. They know it's every two hours, and every two hours on the dot they'll let you know it's been two hours. Their pain is always a 10. They're always hungry. I'll get an extra meal tray for them. Once they're better, got some drugs, food, they leave against medical advice. As if they want to get back to the streets, their home. Anthony King came in last March—it's July now—was here for two days, and left against medical advice. He told me he didn't have any money for the bus. He was Native. He could be surly. I gave him 10 bucks. Discharges usually go out in a wheelchair. We have a transport person—Colleen—whom you can call, but I always walk them out, even the irascible Anthony. Out of the ICU through Med-Surg to the elevator down to the first floor. I talk to them, ask them where they're going to stay tonight, what their plans are, give them some encouragement. Sometimes they're trying to get into a residential detox. Move in with an aunt. Get a job. I always walk them outside and then say goodbye to them. I walked Anthony to the door of the hospital and, because he was unsteady, walked him to the crosswalk on Montgomery. I watched him walk across Montgomery and walk right past the bus stop on his way to Smith's to get a bottle. I haven't seen him since.

Leo Tolstoy wrote that his idea of happiness was "a quiet secluded life in the country, with the possibility of being useful to people to whom it is easy to do good, and who are not accustomed to have it done to them; then work which one hopes may be of some use; then rest, nature, books, music, love for one's neighbor."[19] I know they're not accustomed to have someone do good to them, their daily life is a rebuke, but I feel fortunate to be in a position to be able to do something for them that requires so little of me—just a few words, a sandwich, a bag of chips, a few bucks—so for a while they don't feel that they're outcasts exiled from the human family, that they fell from a ship into waters where they'll eventually drown some dark night; so that they know they may be on a hard road but they're still sacred souls.

13

Achilles in Vietnam

I work three days, have five off, then three. Patients come and go whom you never see. Or maybe they leave the first day you're back so you never take care of them. His name is Christopher Esteban. I don't know him. He's ICU status. He's in room 225. It's a negative-pressure room to rule out tuberculosis, so it has an anteroom the size of a walk-in closet where you gown up and put on your PAPR mask. It's a powered air purifying respirator, which is motorized and delivers filtered air. He had a respiratory event on Med-Surg and was transferred to the ICU. He's on BiPaP (bilevel positive airway pressure). It's a thick plastic face mask strapped around your head to make as tight a seal as possible. It's attached to a machine by a thick plastic hose. It's for patients in respiratory failure. It pushes air into your lungs, opens them up. There's pressure throughout the breathing cycle, high when you inhale, lower when you exhale. It's loud. A patient said to me it's like having a hurricane on your face. You can't eat or drink on BiPAP. It's also called noninvasive ventilation because if you fail BiPAP, the next step is a ventilator. He had been weaned off it on days but required it at night.

The unit's full. In rounds they always try to see if somebody can be downgraded and move out to Med-Surg to make space for admissions. No one's ready to move out. In the afternoon the house supervisor calls to say a patient in the ER needs an ICU bed. Gavin tells her we have no beds, no one's moving out. We hear the chief nursing officer (CNO) is putting pressure on the hospitalist to downgrade and transfer somebody. He relents and decides to transfer 225. Veronica is the Med-Surg charge today. When she's told who the transfer is, she comes to the ICU to talk to the physician. She knows what happened to the patient on Med-Surg. The nurse calling for help. Finding him sitting up in bed, arms clutching the side rails, struggling to breathe. He had pulled his gown off. They called a REACT. They were lucky to get him to the ICU. She tells the physician she doesn't think he should be transferred. She was told no one was moving out. Why did he change his mind? The CNO comes into the unit to find out why the patient hasn't been transferred. The physician leaves and walks away into another patient's room. Veronica tells the CNO she doesn't feel it's safe to transfer him back to Med-Surg. She feels she doesn't have qualified staff to take care of him. That he would be at risk on Med-Surg. Veronica's opposed to the transfer but not because he would be a busy patient, a burden to her unit. It's called advocacy. Veronica is advocating for the patient.

In their early pilot work on the role of intuition in clinical judgment and later in their study of the development of expertise in critical care nursing practice, nurse scholars Patricia Benner and Christine Tanner noticed a recurring discourse among nurses about "knowing the patient." This led to a 1993 study, "The Phenomenology of Knowing the Patient," published in the *Journal of Nursing Scholarship*, where Tanner, Benner, and colleagues interviewed 130 nurses who practiced in adult, pediatric, and newborn ICUs of eight hospitals in three metropolitan areas. Two kinds of knowing the patient emerged from the study: knowing the patient's patterns of responses and knowing the patient as a person.[1]

Knowing the patient isn't a matter of friendliness or personal intimacy. Knowing the patient is a professional, not a personal, relationship. It means knowing the patient's reaction to treatments and medications, coping resources, progress; being attuned to the patient's suffering, concerns, resourcefulness, and possibilities. Knowing is central to skilled clinical judgment. It leads to expert nursing practice. Knowing enables the nurse to recognize clinical changes and leads to patient-centered responses. Tanner and colleagues define it as "tacit embodied, [sic] know-how that allows for the instantaneous recognition of patterns and intuitive responses."[2] It also leads to advocacy.

The nurses in the study saw themselves as advocates who stand alongside patients and their families when they are weak and vulnerable. They talked about their commitment to be vigilant and ensure that appropriate care is given. A 2019 study published in the journal *Nursing Ethics* identified several characteristics of nursing advocacy: "Apprising" provides patients with information regarding their diagnoses, prognoses, and treatments. "Mediating" is acting as a liaison for patients with other health-care professionals, being their voice if necessary. "Safeguarding" protects patients if other health-care professionals aren't competent or have committed misconduct. "Valuing" ensures patients are able to make decisions freely and have a right to privacy, and it acknowledges patients' beliefs and cultural values.[3]

The Hippocratic oath is an oath of ethics historically taken by physicians. It requires a new physician to swear, by a number of healing gods, to uphold specific ethical standards such as medical confidentiality and nonmaleficence. Nurses don't take a comparable oath, but the American Nurses Association does have a Code of Ethics for Nurses. It contains provisions that are directly related to nursing advocacy: Provision 2 states that nurses' primary commitment is to their patients and requires nurses to provide patients with the opportunity to participate in the development of treatment plans. Provision 3 obligates nurses to protect and advocate for patients' safety, rights, and health.[4]

Advocacy is being the patients' voice, speaking for them when they are unable to do so, whether by medical condition, education, cultural difference, or exclusion from participation in treatment plans or medical decisions. Advocacy might be asking for another day of weaning the ventilator before doing a tracheostomy. It might be advocating for palliative care. Or asking not to transfer the patient out of the ICU because he's not ready.

The nursing station ends across from 226. Veronica and the CNO are facing each other. It's a standoff. Veronica says the policy is that patients on BiPAP for the first time can't go to Med-Surg. The CNO says, "Show me the policy." Veronica asks why the ER patient can't go to another hospital. When a hospital is unable to admit a patient because its beds are full, the patient is "diverted" to a facility that has available beds. It's standard practice among Albuquerque hospitals. Before Ventas bought Ardent, it was our policy. The CNO doesn't say anything. Usually when the physician decides to transfer your patient out of the ICU, you agree. Labs are good. The chest film is clear. You've advanced the diet. But you might not. She spiked a temp. Her pain's not well controlled. It doesn't feel like she's ready. The physician will listen. You'll talk about it. She might not change her mind, but maybe she'll repeat a lab. Transfer the patient as Intermediate Care status, not Med-Surg, so there's closer monitoring. Or tell you why it's OK. It's a dialogue. This isn't a dialogue. It's not really a standoff because the CNO wins.

When the patient's sister hears he's being transferred back to Med-Surg, she's distraught. She doesn't understand why he's leaving the ICU. She doesn't want him to be transferred. No one told her that might happen. Not the physician in the morning. Not the nurse. He leaves the ICU just before shift change. His room in Med-Surg is blocked off so the sister can stay with him overnight. He's on telemetry, monitored in the ICU. It's early the next morning. The sister is asleep in the adjacent bed. The Med-Surg nurse goes into the room to check on him. He's blue. His BiPAP is off. They code him. He doesn't respond. They call the code. They call the ICU and ask the monitor tech to run a six-second strip. The tech tells the nurse he's in sinus rhythm on the monitor. They bring him to the ICU and continue the code. His sister is screaming, "I'm going to sue." It's futile. He's dead.

The next morning at shift change, Veronica is on the elevator to the second floor. The door opens and the night supervisor is waiting to get on. The supervisor is pushing an opened crash cart. "Rough night?" She tells her who. The supervisor had recently given her notice and was working her final shifts. "I'm done," she says. "I'm not coming back." A few months later, Veronica resigned. "I got into nursing to help people," she told me. Later that day the hospitalist says to me, "If he was still in the ICU, he'd be alive today." For several days after the death, the CNO was in the ICU with IT adjusting the alarms on the monitors, lowering the thresholds, as if the alarms had something to do with his death.

Tanner and colleagues write, "When nurses work in situations where it is impossible to protect patients from violation of patient and family concerns or threats to their vulnerability, then the very ground for safe and astute nursing care is undermined. In such situations, nursing loses its ground as a practice with notions of good internal to it."[5]

In the early 1980s, the philosopher Andrew Jameton, who taught about ethical issues in health care, was having a classroom discussion with a group of nurses on bioethical dilemmas such as appropriate care for dying patients and limits to life support. The nurses responded with heartfelt stories in which they recalled with deep regret situations where they were required to perform not just futile care but uncomfortable or painful procedures on patients for whom there was no hope for cure.

Traditional bioethics focuses on ethical dilemmas where the lone practitioner must choose between two ethically justifiable but mutually opposing actions. Bioethics texts appeal to abstract moral theories. Decisions are made by cognitive reasoning. Jameton felt what the nurses revealed to him was the emotional side of ethical dilemmas.

Jameton's experience led to his 1984 book, *Nursing Practice: The Ethical Issues*, which introduced the concept of moral distress to nursing.[6] Moral distress is defined as the experience of knowing the right thing to do while being constrained from doing it. Unlike ethical dilemmas, moral distress doesn't involve a difficulty in choosing between alternatives; the nurse has moral certainty—knows the morally correct action to take—but is unable to do it. A key element in moral distress is the sense of powerlessness.

The constraints are often institutional policies and practices: short-staffing, inadequately trained staff, power imbalances between members of the health-care team, cost containment, lack of administrative support. Some of these problems are specific to the institutions in which nurses work; broader factors are related to challenges of the health-care system, corporate ownership, or profit-oriented management.

The course of illness is rife with ethical issues. There are forks in the road every day. Intubate? Extubate? Feed? Paralyze? You have to decide which one to take. Communicating with families is a seesaw of hope and truth. Nursing is negotiating, sometimes clashing, with physicians. Most nurses don't experience significant distress from difficult situations at work. They have moral resilience. Moral resilience is the ability to sustain your integrity, your ethical balance. Resilience comes from experience, the recognition of limits, the belief you've done the best you could do in the circumstance. You learn how to navigate through discord, conflict, uncertainty. When to stand your ground. When to take a step back. When to let go.

Moral injury is different.

The term "moral injury" originated in the 1990s in the writings of physician and clinical psychiatrist Jonathan Shay, author of *Achilles in Vietnam: Combat Trauma and the Undoing of Character*.[7] The book is based on the memories of his patients who were Vietnam veterans and their experience of leadership malpractice. "Shay's definition of moral injury has three components: 'Moral injury is present when (i) there has been a betrayal of what is morally right, (ii) by someone who holds legitimate authority (iii) in a high-stakes situation.'"[8]

In "The Closure of Hahnemann University Hospital and the Experience of Moral Injury in Academic Medicine," physician Laura Weiss Roberts writes of the loss felt by patients, faculty, staff, and neighboring communities when the Philadelphia hospital closed. Echoing Shay's definition, she writes that moral injury is a betrayal of what is right by people in a position of trust, in a situation of consequence: "Moral injury is when we experience a rupture in how things ought to be, a sense that those with authentic and legitimate authority have acted in a manner that lacks integrity or have failed to preserve or protect things that truly matter."[9] The thing that truly mattered to her was the integrity of academic medicine. Academic medical centers are not only teaching hospitals; they provide care for underserved populations and communities. The abrupt closure of Hahnemann meant the end of a safety net hospital that had provided care for the vulnerable and poor of central Philadelphia for decades, a population to which the field of academic medicine is uniquely devoted.

Sentinel Event Alert 57's focus on the role of leadership in creating a safety culture emphasized not only policy measures but personal conduct. Culture is a product of what is done on a daily basis. Hospital employees measure an organization's commitment to safety culture by a leader's everyday actions, decisions, and behaviors. The alert called for all leaders, from CEOs to managers, to model appropriate behaviors and champion efforts to eradicate intimidating behaviors. These behaviors include demonstrating respect in all interactions and making sure safety-related feedback from staff is acknowledged and, if appropriate, implemented.

The Institute of Medicine has identified the importance of non-hierarchical decision-making as a key element of patient safety. In his writings on shared governance, Tim Porter-O'Grady says, "In today's world of transformative health care and the changing technological framework for practice, there is simply no way that nurses can continue in hierarchical and professionally passive organizational configurations."[10] Shared governance has been a driving force in the transformation of the hierarchical structure of hospitals and the increase in the clinical decision-making role of nurses.

Echoing the Joint Commission's sentinel event alert on leadership, Porter-O'Grady emphasizes the role of leadership in implementing and sustaining shared governance. Leadership is instrumental in helping staff develop competence in making decisions on issues of practice and creating a safe environment so that trials and issues associated with changes in power dynamics and traditional locus of control can be safely navigated.

Private equity's success in co-opting leaders by offering financial incentives and aligning their behavior and values with the goals of the private equity company severs their relationship with staff, abrogates the commitment to safety, and betrays the presumption of a shared mission. The cultural change promised in shared governance is undermined, and the realignment leads to a betrayal of what is morally right and a failure to protect the thing that truly matters: the welfare of the patient.

In January 2021, Brigham and Women's Hospital announced that Elizabeth Nabel was resigning after 11 years as CEO effective March 1. Her resignation followed 2020 allegations by the *Boston Globe*'s investigative journalism unit, Spotlight, that since 2015 Nabel had served on the board of Moderna, the manufacturer of a COVID-19 vaccine that was being tested in a nationwide trial. Brigham and Women's Hospital was one of 89 clinical trial sites participating in the phase-three trial of the vaccine. After the *Globe* asked hospital officials whether Nabel's position at the biotech firm was a conflict of interest with her hospital's work in the clinical trial, she resigned from the Moderna board on July 30, 2020.[11]

According to the *Globe*, which cites information filed with the Securities and Exchange Commission, Dr. Nabel sold millions of dollars in Moderna stock before her resignation from the board. She "sold 30,000 shares . . . worth $1.98 million in May and 73,975 . . . shares worth $6.5 million on July 15," after the company's stock nearly quadrupled that year in light of news of early success with its experimental COVID-19 vaccine, "bringing her total earnings this year [2020] to about $8.5 million."[12]

A number of Brigham and Women's employees were angered by Nabel's profit from the stock sales because it coincided with the hospital's cost-cutting due to COVID-19. In a June 17 email to the employees, Nabel said the hospital's parent company, Mass General Brigham, was cutting executive pay, freezing salaries of other employees, and suspending contributions to their retirement plan because of the financial damage from the pandemic.

On August 24, 2020, a month after Nabel's resignation from the Moderna board, the *Globe* published an editorial: "Hospitals Need a Stronger Prescription for Keeping the Public's Trust." The editorial quotes Charles Binkley, director of bioethics at the Markkula Center for Applied Ethics at Santa Clara University: "A hospital leader has different moral obligations. It's impossible to meet those moral obligations when you are also a board member with a fiduciary responsibility to propel the profits of a company—not to mention the opportunity to enrich yourself from those company profits." The editorial concludes with this statement: "Hospitals are special places, and their leaders have special obligations. One of those obligations is absolute, undiluted loyalty to the community they lead and serve. That includes patients and their families, along with the entire universe of hospital employees—from doctors, nurses and nurse's aides to cleaning crews and cafeteria staff."[13]

14

Promises

It's just before six in the evening. Gavin sticks a yellow Post-it to the top corner of my computer. David Yazzie. 32. GIB.

"From Gallup," he says. "They're in the air."

Ten minutes later, the nurse from Gallup calls to give me report. History of alcoholism. Massive gastrointestinal bleed (GIB). Bright red blood orally and rectally. Intubated. Transfused with four packed red blood cells and two fresh frozen plasmas. Potassium 2.1.

I get the room ready. Two suctions. A Yankauer. An Ambu bag. Zero the bed. Extra chux. Three pumps. He'll need blood, so I prime some blood tubing with normal saline. On the roller table I put an MRSA swab, gown, clothing bag, thermometer. The EKG cables are hanging loose from the metal ceiling pole like vines.

He comes at shift change. Three EMS guys in bulky yellow-and-black uniforms pushing the stretcher. They wheel the stretcher into the room. It's like the confluence of two rivers. The EMTs, three of us, the bed, the stretcher, the vent, the pumps. But we're like a dance troupe. We know the choreography. Line up and lift him from the stretcher to the bed. Pass bags of fluid. Connect tubing. Voices in the air. His last systolic was 82. Dopamine's at 20. He's got an 18 in the right forearm and a 16 in the left antecubital. Kristen opens the nasogastric tube to suction and turns her head away at the same time. "Can someone get me a mask with a shield?" Temp 35.8. Any family with him? Hearing "him" makes me look at the bed. On both sides of his face are towels that were white but now are blood soaked. Dried black blood flakes on his face. Blood is matted in his hair, on his gown. Like he was rescued from a fire of blood. Nights takes over. On the way out, Gavin asks me, "You back?" I nod and he says, "I wonder if he'll be here."

I can tell he's alive in the morning because the overhead lights in the unit are dimmed like they do on nights but his room is brightly lit like the one room in a dark house where a parent has been up all night with a sick child. The glass doors are wide open off their tracks. The crash cart is in the room, all the drawers open. On the board next to his name, it says 1:1. He would be my only patient.

The room looks storm lashed, but it's not leaves or branches that are strewn about but boxes of epinephrine, bicarb, saline flush wrappers, EKG strips, and empty plastic bags, some with red droplets of packed cells or yellow droplets of plasma. The night nurse gives me report. He coded twice. They got him back both times. He's on the massive transfusion protocol. It's the rapid administration of large amounts of blood products. For every unit of packed red blood cells, you give one unit of fresh frozen plasma. For every six units of red blood cells, you give one unit of platelets. It's called the 1:1:1 ratio. You would give six units of red blood cells, six units of FFP, and one unit of platelets.

The portal vein is a blood vessel that delivers blood to the liver from the stomach, intestines, spleen, and pancreas. Scarring of the liver from cirrhosis causes resistance to the blood flow. It's called portal hypertension. The increased pressure goes as far back as the esophagus. Esophageal veins have thin walls and are close to the surface. Swollen esophageal veins are called varices.

If the pressure in the veins gets too high, they bleed. Varices can also develop in the small blood vessels in the upper part of the stomach. Gastrointestinal bleeding is an emergency. You can bleed out. The treatment is an esophagogastroduodenoscopy (EGD). It's also called an upper endoscopy. It's a procedure where the physician threads a thin scope with a light and camera at the tip through the patient's mouth to look at the esophagus, the stomach, and the first part of the small intestine. You watch it on a monitor the size of a small TV. There's a banding device attached to the tip of the endoscope. When you find the vein that's bleeding, you pull it into a chamber where a trip wire dislodges a rubber band and ties off the trapped vein. The nurse said his pressure was soft so they couldn't sedate him, and when the GI doc inserted the scope, the patient moved, so he stopped. They were going to try again today. She gave me report in the room where she was charting on her computer. Another nurse was helping her. There's a lot of documentation when you give blood. She was way behind. At ten o'clock that morning she was still in the unit charting.

He has an arterial line so it's real-time blood pressure. He's on 12 of Levophed. His systolic is in the low 100s. No gown. Two white defibrillator pads on his chest. He's not sedated. When they're sedated it's like they're submerged, but he's not. He's right there, like a needle on the skin of water. Opens his eyes, shows two fingers. I think he's brave to lie there awake, still, quiet. What was it like to leave and come back twice last night? He's alive but the trapdoor he fell through twice last night is still open. I think what they could have done. If he's actively bleeding like he was, you have to find the source. They could have sedated him a little more with some propofol. Put him on another pressor. Give him some albumin or Hespan to pump up his blood pressure. If you're good and lucky, it could only take 5, 10 minutes. Find it. Band it. In and out. If he was the son of the CEO, would they have said, "Okay. He moved. We'll do it tomorrow"? Dying while Navajo.

You can think of them as a tragic, ruined people. Navajo Nation is a remote wasteland of no running water, dirt roads, poverty, alcoholism. But then you think about what they've survived, all the attempts to destroy their culture. In 1864, Kit Carson, working for the US Army, launched an assault on the Navajo. His goal was to eradicate their way of life. Carson burned hogans to the ground, slaughtered livestock, destroyed irrigated fields. The Navajo who surrendered were taken to Fort Canby. Those who resisted were murdered. Then the Long Walk. In 1864 when the Navajo refused to accept confinement on reservations, Carson marched more than 8,500 men, women, and children 400 miles across New Mexico in the dead of winter at gunpoint for imprisonment on the Bosque Redondo Reservation, where the military maintained an outpost. The journey lasted 18 days. Hundreds died of starvation and exposure. The purpose was to forcibly change the Navajo from a nomadic to an agricultural tribe. In 1868, after four years on the disease-ridden reservation, surrounded by enemy troops, starving on meager rations, the Navajo signed the Treaty of Bosque Redondo, which ended their incarceration on the Bosque Redondo Reservation. On June 18, 1868, the Navajo began the long walk home.

Livestock was the foundation of the Navajo economy during the first quarter of the twentieth century. The average Navajo family owned 100 head of horses, 300 head of sheep, and 100 head of cattle. The Navajo had deep cultural and spiritual ties to their herds. They believed livestock was given to them by the Holy People. Navajo would sing over their flocks, corrals, and the lands where the animals grazed. The Navajo practiced a nomadic pastoralism that anthropologists called transhumance, a seasonal movement of flocks to higher pastures in the summer and lower valleys in the winter. Grazing is fundamental to Navajo identity. In the 1930s, the US government claimed that grazing areas were becoming eroded from too many animals. In what is known as the

Navajo Livestock Reduction, the federal government killed more than 80% of Navajo livestock. Starting in 1933, the goat herds were the first to be gathered and killed. A year later, the sheep were killed, followed by horses and cattle. Federal agents would sometimes kill the animals in front of grieving families. By the time the reduction had run its course between 1933 and 1946, the Navajo economy was devastated. Impoverishment and dependence on the government became a part of reservation life. The Navajo refer to these events as the Second Long Walk.[1]

A family conference had been planned for the morning. We meet in the NICU conference room on the second floor at eight. There are maybe 20 family members. They're not related like Anglos are, not brothers or sisters in the way Anglos are. There are 60 Navajo clans. They have names like Poles-Strung-Out, Under-His-Cover, Who-Encircles-One, Trail-to-the-Garden. Each clan is associated with from one to six other clans. All members of your clan and of the clans linked to yours are considered "sisters," "brothers," "fathers." To a Navajo, relatives are the most important thing. The Navajo say, "Act as if everybody were related to you."[2]

There are long tables along the back and side walls with metal folding chairs on one side facing into the room. The Navajo distance themselves so there's someone at each table. Dr. Chapman is the pulmonologist today. He's standing, facing them, with his back to a pulled-down white projector screen. Gail, the GI nurse practitioner, is next to him.

Chapman begins by talking about what happened last night, the EGD they couldn't do, that his heart had stopped twice, that his condition was serious, the plans for an EGD today. He then asks, if his heart were to stop again, would they want him to be resuscitated or would they just want "to let him go"? They are as still as the mesas that dot the Navajo reservation, but then someone says, like a breeze that stirs the leaves of a tree but so slightly you can't tell where it came from, "Let him go." Then others say,

"Let him go." Chapman then says it's important to know "what David would want." He asks if anyone knows what David would want in this situation. His wife is sitting at the end of the first table when you enter the room. Her name is Erika. She has tissues in both of her hands. Her head is down. "He wouldn't want to go through it again." She doesn't look up. Chapman then asks, in the event it happened, would members of the family want to be with him as he passed away? And then he asks who would want to be with him. Each of them either nods or raises a hand. He thanks the family and leaves. I go over to where his wife is sitting. I get down on one knee to be close to her. I say, "Erika, just to be sure, if he has any life-threatening event, we're not going to do any chest compressions or shock him, we're going to let him go?"

"Yes."

"So he'll be a Do Not Resuscitate. Until that happens, we'll do everything we can for him. Our nurses worked hard to keep him alive last night. Many of them are still here. And we'll do the same today. But if that moment comes, we'll let him go. And you can be with him." In the ICU, when you reach this point, make this decision, you have to be sure everyone understands, everyone agrees. It's like staking a tent to the ground. You want to be sure everything is in place, that everything is secure, when the storm comes.

I call the GI lab at nine to see when they plan on doing the EGD. They say they're doing cases. They say the same thing at ten. The lab is on the same floor as the ICU. You walk through Med-Surg across an overlook to the lobby. The door is locked. There's a phone on the wall. A nurse opens the door. I tell her the patient coded twice last night and whatever's on their schedule, they need to bump it and scope him. "We're finishing up," she says.

He can only get 2.5 milligrams of Versed every 4 hours and 25–50 of fentanyl every 30 minutes. It's not enough to fully sedate him for the procedure, so I go to the side of the bed and tell him what we're going to do and that it's very important that he not move when they insert the scope. His eyes are closed. With his right hand, he gives me a thumbs up. I put my hand flat on his chest over his heart. "You're a warrior." They do the EGD just after eleven. Alvarez is the GI doc. He can't find it. There are no esophageal varices bleeding, and when he gets to the stomach, it's full of blood. He pulls out the scope. He wants to repeat the EGD in two hours with a larger tube from Lovelace Medical Center.

It's two hours later. The tube is an Ewald tube to lavage the stomach. It's a large bore, a 30 French. You need to wash out the blood and clots to see the gastric varices. Suction canisters can hold up to one liter, 1,000 ccs of fluid. I had already replaced one and the second one was filling up. I had to call out for someone to bring more canisters. Alvarez is twisting the tip of the probe along the folds of the stomach. There's blood everywhere. He's talking as he works. "C'mon, where are you?" All of a sudden there it is. Like stalking a ship in a fog and the fog lifts and there it is. "It's a gastric varix." In 1969 Mark Rothko painted a three-by-two-foot oil on paper mounted on canvas. It was two large red rectangles against a red background. It was titled *Red on Red*. The screen looks like that. He tries to band it. The bands won't hold. Every time he tries, it bleeds again. I've seen it only once before. At St. Vincent in Santa Fe. It was the same thing. A bedside EGD. A nurse yelling, "I need help!" The monitor all blood. A code. He died. It looks like that.

"I can't get it." He pulls out the scope. The screen goes dark. "I'll talk to the family." The third suction canister is full.

A woman comes into the room. Silver-buttoned calico blouse. Pleated velveteen skirt. A shawl over her shoulders. Her hair in the traditional bun known as a *tsiiyeel* in Navajo. The beauty of the matriarchs. She walks by me quietly and sits in a chair by the window and looks at the bed. She was sitting next to his wife in the morning meeting. Alvarez comes back and tells me the family wants to withdraw support.

Dr. Chapman is in the unit sitting at a computer near Maria. I suddenly hear her say to him loudly, "He's bradying down!" I look at the monitor. His heart rate had been fast all day, in the 130s, trying to push his oxygen-poor blood to the frontiers of his body. Now it's 66, 58, 50. The trapdoor. He's going. A warrior coming to the end. Chapman comes into the room and says, "Give him epi." I turn to him. "He's a DNR. They want to let him go." He barks at me, "Give him epi and get the crash cart." I hear an overhead page, "Code blue, ICU." The room is filling with people. Kristen brings the crash cart, cracks open the plastic lock. Someone tells the woman sitting in the chair, "You have to leave." She says she wants to stay. The person says, "You can't stay."

His chest gives easily to compressions from ribs broken in the earlier codes. Chapman is giving orders. He says give two units of blood. "I want it on a pressure bag, not on a pump. Squeeze it. I want that through the cordis in five minutes." He orders atropine, which is not in the algorithm for cardiac arrest. Everyone knows what to do. That we give epi every three minutes, do CPR to circulate it, then do a rhythm check. We give him epi twice. Sodium bicarb. Two units of blood. People rotate doing compressions. After you've given them epi, compressions, someone will do a pulse check and you'll hear, "Bounding carotid." But we check and there's no pulse. No pressure. I put the Levo at 30. The ER charge had come to the code. A young nurse came with her. She was standing behind me. "What's your max on Levo?" she whispers.

"Twenty if they're alive. Thirty if they're dead."

Codes can feel heroic at first, as if the patient has just slipped below the surface of the water and you can reach into the water and get ahold of a hand or an arm and pull them up, but then you've given a round of drugs and you do a rhythm check and it's a flat line and then another round of drugs and there's no pulse and you realize they're beyond your reach deep below the surface, where light doesn't reach, drifting down, and you've crossed a line and it doesn't feel heroic; it feels cruel and wrong; and then someone will ask, "Should we stop?" and then someone will say, "I think we should stop," and finally the physician will ask if anyone has any objections to calling the code and no one does and the physician calls the code.

The blood is in. The advanced cardiac life support drugs are in. No rhythm. The room's quiet. We've crossed that line. Gavin's doing CPR. We're waiting. There's talk during a code. Someone will ask when was the last epi. If there's a pulse with compressions. If the person doing CPR wants to switch. Silence is a message. Finally, Chapman asks, "Are there any objections to calling the code?" There are no objections.

We clean his face, put a fresh gown on him, take out the endotracheal tube, and let the family in. They huddle around the bed. Most of the pueblo Indians speak Keres. Keres sounds like a foreign language, but familiar, like Spanish or Italian. Navajo is like no other language. The anthropologist Clyde Kluckhohn describes it as having a nonchalant, mechanical flavor, almost as if a robot were talking. The same word can have a different meaning with a small clutch of breath linguists call glottal closure. It can't be learned.

When someone dies, the family has to choose a funeral home to take the body. We give them a list of homes in Albuquerque. If they don't pick one, the body goes to the morgue until they do. Not the Navajo. They're a sovereign nation. "Sovereignty" isn't a Navajo word. The closest word in Dine is *Onni 'Inteego.* "Self-responsibility." Navajo Sovereignty Day is the fourth Monday in April and celebrates the day the Navajo signed the Treaty of Bosque Redondo and gained their independence from the US government. One time in Santa Fe, a family took a patient home to Navajo Nation in the back of a pickup truck. I talk to Erika about picking a funeral home. I tell her that, if they want, they can take him home themselves. But they make some calls and find a service that will take him to Gallup.

The funeral service sends a young man maybe in his 20s. He introduces himself to Erika. Has her sign a few papers. He tells her he's sorry for her loss. The stretcher he's brought has a low metal bed you put a top on with drapes that hide the body. The Navajo follow it as it leaves the unit. They walk behind slowly, processionally, as if they were carrying something sacred but the sacred thing they're carrying is their very selves. Something ancient and pure and never again.

If they don't know you, Navajo won't look you in the eye. They'll look at your ear, your mouth, over your shoulder. They don't like to shake hands. If they do, it's limp. I'm standing just outside the room as they pass by. Erika is the last to leave. She stops in front of me. She extends her hand. I take it. She holds it, looks straight at me, and says she wants to thank me for everything we did. Two women near her say thank you as well.

The Treaty of Bosque Redondo promised each Navajo family 160 acres of land to farm, seeds and agricultural implements for the first year, clothing and raw materials to make clothing for the next 10 years. It promised 15,000 sheep and goats, 500 beef cattle, and 1 million pounds of corn. None of the promises were kept. The land was desert, without water, not arable. The food, clothing, seeds, and tools never came. The Navajo would wait in line for rations. By the end of the first year, they were on the brink of starvation. They're a people used to broken promises.

In a 1968 interview for the book *Navajo Stories of the Long Walk Period*, Howard Gorman, a Dine elder whose ancestors were on the Long Walk, said, "Our ancestors were taken captive and driven to Hwéeldi (the Bosque) for no reason at all. They were harmless people, and, even to date, we are the same, holding no harm for anybody. Many Navajo who know our history and the story of Hwéeldi say the same."[3]

They hold no harm to this day. I failed them and they held me no harm.

After, I played it back. The day. The family conference. "Let him go." The wife. The promise. "You're a warrior." The EGD. All the blood. The family wants to withdraw. The code. Someone kicking that woman out. Dying. I tried to understand what happened when Chapman said to get the crash cart and give epi. What I was thinking. Why I let it happen. I thought of other things I could have done. I could have said, "No, he's a DNR." Stood my ground. I could have asked if his code status had changed. I could have had Maria find his wife and ask her what she wanted to do. I didn't do any of those things. I didn't do what I was supposed to do. I didn't protect him. It wasn't like me. I broke a promise to his wife that he would die peacefully and the family would be with him.

The moment. Every ICU nurse knows it. It's what you train for. To be ready. I heard an interview on NPR with two ICU nurses. They were best friends. They were describing their ICU, the kind of patients they had. They were sharp. You could feel the warmth between them. The interviewer asked them what it was like to work with such sick patients, and one of them said, "No one's dying until they are. And when they do, we're ready." When the moment comes, you're not overwhelmed by it. You make the right decision. I heard a musician talk about what it felt like to have talent. You reach for it and it's there. Beginning in the Neuro ICU at the University of New Mexico Hospital, I watched, I learned, I saw what other nurses did, then I went out into the world and I reached a point where I was ready. When the moment happened, I would reach for it and it would be there. This time, I reached for it and it wasn't there. The moment came and I wasn't ready.

In 1993, Andrew Jameton wrote that not only was there an initial acute experience of moral distress, there was what he called a reactive distress that remained. Subsequent researchers redefined it as moral residue.[4] It's cumulative. The experience of seeing more suffering and death than what is expected, witnessing acts that conflict with deeply held beliefs and values, has long-lasting consequences. Each time a morally distressing situation occurs, the level of moral residue rises. It's called the crescendo effect. It causes damage over time. It can lead to a breaking point. The literature on moral distress talks about the loss of moral compass and moral disorientation, about the disequilibrium it can cause: the feeling of being unable to be yourself in a situation in which you feel that you should but are not able to do the right thing, when "we have seriously compromised ourselves or allowed ourselves to be compromised."[5]

I thought about all that had happened in the last 14 months. The look on that woman's face: "Save me." The card from her children. Pam's father. The woman dying in the elevator. The patient dead and no one knew. The young Navajo mother. The sister screaming. You think what matters is you caring for your patients, doing your best every day, and whether your hospital is a nonprofit or a for-profit or if it's owned by a private equity firm has nothing to do with you. Then it does. Doing things we shouldn't do. Not doing things we should do. If they had brought that patient to the ICU sooner, she would be back in Socorro. If they had given us a sitter, that Navajo mother would be with her children in a hogan. If they hadn't transferred that patient to Med-Surg, he would be home today. Simone Weil wrote, "At the bottom of the heart of every human being, from earliest infancy until the tomb, there is something that goes on indomitably expecting that good and not evil will be done to him. It is this above all that is sacred in every human being."[6] I think each of them came to Lovelace Women's Hospital expecting good would be done to them. And it wasn't. I wondered if they added up. The deaths. If it changed me. The way water will scour a riverbank, erode it over time, until something happens and the riverbank fails. The crescendo effect.

The next morning, Chapman was in the unit. He was sitting in the nurses' station at a computer. I walked over and stood behind the computer facing him and asked why we coded the patient when he was a DNR. Without looking away from the screen, he said, "Viable. Survived two codes."

MIDAS is an online incident-reporting system that "enables hospital staff to submit incident reports of patient safety issues for analysis and improvement."[7] It should trigger an investigation. I filed a MIDAS report and also requested a root cause analysis of why we coded a patient with DNR orders and contrary to the wishes of the family. I gave it to the ICU nurse manager. I wrote that I felt I was remiss in not challenging the physician's order, not clarifying why we were coding a patient who was a DNR. What the family wanted to happen did not happen; and what they didn't want to happen happened. They were not with him, by his side, as he died; and he died the gruesome death of a failed resuscitation.

I wrote that I felt a root cause analysis was necessary not only to understand why a DNR order that had been established with the family was contravened but to illuminate a path of improved physician-nurse communication, especially in high-intensity situations, in order that we could provide appropriate patient-centered care. And keep our promise.

15

Pentimento

Sue Bowes was a registered nurse who had worked at Hahnemann for 14 years. She was also president of the local chapter of the Pennsylvania Association of Staff Nurses and Allied Professionals union. When the 171-year-old hospital closed, she had a message for other communities around the United States where private equity firms were buying hospitals: "Be scared."[1] She had high hopes when the private equity firm Paladin Healthcare bought the hospital and promised changes and improvements. Paladin's president, Barry Wolfman, had stated that the company's goal was "to return Hahnemann to its rightful place in the landscape of healthcare."[2] But those hopes disappeared when Hahnemann announced its planned closure amid reports the property would be redeveloped as luxury condos. The lesson Bowes learned was that the financial goals of private equity firms don't align with the mission of a hospital or the values of the people who work in one.

I never received a response to my MIDAS report or to my request for a root cause analysis. The leadership at Lovelace Women's Hospital was in flux. The ICU manager I gave it to had resigned. We received an internal email that the chief nursing officer (CNO) had resigned and transferred to quality. The ER manger left. There was an interim CNO. An interim ICU manager. They weren't from New Mexico. There were rumors. That there was a class action suit for wrongful deaths. That there were meetings about the patient from 225 about mandatory nondisclosure. That the CNO was kept as an employee because of Ardent's policy prohibiting employees from speaking to the press.

I was charge one day. Seven patients and only two nurses. The night charge apologized. She said she tried to get me a nurse or even a tech but administration said no. I called the house supervisor and told her I wasn't accepting the shift until we got another nurse. Being an ICU nurse means having the confidence that whatever comes through the door, you'll be able to handle it. It's a confidence that comes from experience, skill, necessity. Now it felt like there could be a situation that we wouldn't be able to handle, that would be overwhelming. A code on the floor, a patient deteriorating in the unit at the same time. Not enough staff. Be scared.

Daniela came to the ICU as a young nurse from Med-Surg three years ago. She's in her late 20s. An Albuquerque girl. Two young children. Husband a police officer. After a year she moved to San Diego to help care for an ailing relative. She worked in a burn unit at a Level 1 trauma. She came back six months ago. She was a good nurse when she left. She was a great nurse when she came back. You think of nurses like Daniela and Kristen as the future, the next generation of critical care nurses at Women's. One day Daniela told me she wanted to ask me a question. We went into the break room. It took her a few seconds. She told me that something felt wrong. She thought that we would always have the best plan. That we would always support the patient. Do what's right. We weren't doing that. It didn't feel safe. Things had changed. "What happens when you leave or when Gavin leaves?" She told me she was thinking of transferring to Presbyterian and asked what I thought she should do. When she was finished, she looked down. I wondered for a second if she was afraid I would be disappointed in her. I told her right away that she should go. That things had changed. That something could happen that she would have no control over, and it could affect her license and her career. I told her how much I respected her. How much confidence I had in her. That she was going to have a wonderful career. Presbyterian would be a great opportunity. She looked relieved. She smiled kind of sadly and told me it felt like the boiling frog story: If you put a frog in a pot of boiling water, it will jump out right away. But if you put it in warm water, and turn the heat up slowly, it won't sense that it's getting hotter and will stay in the water until it's boiled to death. But she said she felt the water getting warmer.

The patient's name is Stella Cardenas. She's 32. She's in 230. She had been "found down" outside her home with coffee-ground emesis around her mouth and on the ground. EMS brought her in. Her systolic pressure was 72. Her lactate 20. Her hematocrit and hemoglobin 8 and 22. Her liver enzymes elevated. For someone so young, she had a long medical history: alcoholism, hepatitis, PTSD, anxiety, meth, victim of domestic abuse, multiple falls with a traumatic brain injury. She was diagnosed with acute hepatic failure, encephalopathy, gastrointestinal bleeding. They gave her blood and fresh frozen plasma. Put her on a bicarb drip. Started lactulose. On the second day she had a seizure. The head CT was normal. The CT of the chest showed hepatic nodules suspicious for hepatocellular cancer. It's hospital day 3.

In the ICU, you are said to "follow" the nurse who gives you report, like "I followed so-and-so." Some nurses are good to follow. The room is clean, they checked the morning glucose, labs are drawn. Some aren't. The plague of inexperience that began in Med-Surg has reached the ICU. Electrolytes aren't replaced. They don't know the vent settings. Diagnostic tests that were ordered aren't done. EEGs used to be done by a tech from Lovelace Medical Center. When she retired, the hospital trained a few in-house nurses to do them. Some of them weren't good at it. The nurse I followed told me they ordered an EEG but the nurse had a problem with the machine and left without doing it.

I look at the patient's labs. Her pH is corrected but she's still on the bicarb drip. Her potassium is 2.5 and wasn't replaced. Liver enzymes—AST, ALT—are proteins that help your blood clot, break down toxins, fight infection. If your liver is injured, it releases these enzymes into your bloodstream. Hers are sky-high.

In the room are two people. A man is sleeping in one of the big chairs. His head is on a folded white hospital blanket on a roller table cradled in arms covered with tattoos. A baseball cap with an NY logo resting on his head, the bill over his eyes. He looks to be the age of the patient. A woman is standing at the side of the bed looking down at the patient like she has dropped something into a lake and is waiting for it to come up. The mother. She's smoker thin. The skin under one eye is soft and bluish like oyster flesh. It twitches. Then it twitches again. She is wearing jeans, a tucked-in western shirt. Her hair is lusterless like flower petals when they dry. I ask her what the doctors are saying.

"She's sick but stable. They're going to . . ."—she pulls a piece of paper from her shirt pocket—"increase the lactulose and start her on rifampin." That's what yesterday's physician note said. It also said, "Not expected to survive hospital stay." "I cry and pray all the time. I've been waiting for her to come home for twenty years. I'm not going to stop now. She's been lost in drugs. She would come home and sleep and leave. Stay with friends. She had boyfriends. I adopted her son. He has an appointment for speech therapy today. He has a cleft palate. He's three."

I look at her daughter on the bed. A pentimento is a trace of an earlier painting that has been painted over. A painting behind a painting. *The Old Guitarist* is an oil painting by Picasso. Infrared images reveal a different figure hidden behind the old guitarist. The patient's face is gaunt. Her skin pale. Scabs on her cheeks from skin picking. But you can see behind that another image, that she was once beautiful. The image the mother sees.

She's comatose. Encephalopathy is disease or damage that affects the brain. There are several types. Metabolic. Anoxic. Hepatic encephalopathy is from liver disease. It happens when the liver can't process ammonia. Ammonia is a waste product from the digestion of protein. Your body gets rid of it through the liver. With liver failure, ammonia builds up in the blood and then travels to the brain. It's toxic. It can cause confusion, disorientation, coma. Death. Her ammonia had gone from 74 when she first came in to 289 the day she seized. Normal is 15 to 45 µ/dL.

We assess head to toe. I open her eyelids. Her sclera is yellow from jaundice. Her pupils react to light but aren't equal. Left greater than the right by a millimeter. It's called anisocoria. It can be benign, something you have. Like a birthmark. It affects up to 20% of the population. But it can be pathological. A sign of a stroke, bleeding, a tumor. Anisocoria that's new, that you didn't have when you came in, is a neurosurgical emergency because something is putting pressure on the third cranial nerve, causing the pupil to dilate.

The Glasgow Coma Scale was developed in 1974 by the British neurosurgeons Bryan Jennet and Graham Teasdale, who taught at the University of Glasgow Medical School. It was first used by the nursing staff in the Glasgow neurosurgical unit. It's used to measure a person's level of consciousness. It's based on three criteria: eye opening, verbal response, and motor response. A person's score can range from 3 (completely unresponsive) to 15 (completely responsive). Her Glasgow is 4. She gets a 1 for not opening her eyes. A 1 for no verbal response. To assess motor ability, you first ask them to show you two fingers. In the Glasgow that means follows commands. They get a 6 for that. If they can't do that, you see how they respond to pain. You pinch the trapezius muscle that runs between the neck and the shoulder. She did what's called decerebrate posturing. It is also called abnormal extension. The head and neck arch backward. The arms and legs extend. The wrists flex. The feet rotate internally with the toes pointed downward. It can be a symptom of injury to the brainstem or cerebrum. It gives her a 2 on the motor portion of the scale.

The West Haven criteria are considered the gold standard for categorizing the severity of hepatic encephalopathy. They differentiate four grades, from personality changes to lethargy, with each grade having a neurologic symptom like tremors or slurred speech. Grade 4 is coma. The neurologic finding is decerebrate posturing.

The last thing I check is the Babinski reflex. The reflex was described by the neurologist Joseph Babinski in 1896. It's a marker for the health of the cortical spinal tract, which is a nerve channel that sends information between the brain and the spinal cord. It's responsible for motor control in the body and limbs. You stroke the sole of the foot with a blunt object like a tongue depressor or the edge of a key from the heel along the outside edge of the foot toward the big toe. The normal response is for the toes to flex downward toward the source of the stimulus to protect the sole of the foot. The abnormal response, called Babinski's sign, is when the big toe bends up and back to the top of the foot and the other toes fan out. The Babinski reflex is one of the normal reflexes in babies and young children up to 2 years old. It may disappear as early as 12 months. When the Babinski reflex is present in a child older than 2 years or in an adult, it can be a sign of a central nervous system disorder such as brain tumor, meningitis, or stroke.

Epic is our electronic medical record. There's a place to document the Babinski. Most nurses don't do it because it's not something they know. Critical care nurses know cardiology, pulmonary, renal failure. They tend not to know neurology. No one has charted the Babinski on her. I keep a hemostat clamped to my scrub top. It's handy for a lot of things like opening a med vial, clamping a Foley. The tip has a slight curve. I rub it the length of her foot. Her big toe goes up and the others fan out.

She has a medley of neurological signs. They could all be related to her encephalopathy and ammonia levels. But you don't know. They could be missing something. She should be on a ventilator. When we say someone can't protect their airway, we mean they don't have the reflexes to cough or swallow and they're at risk for aspirating and getting pneumonia. Usually a patient with a Glasgow of less than 8 is intubated.

The hospitalist is in the unit sitting in front of a computer. I ask him what the plan is for the patient.

"I'm going to look at the EEG."

"It wasn't done."

"I ordered it yesterday."

"It wasn't done. The nurse couldn't do it."

He's on the phone to the neurologist at Lovelace Medical Center. He's not going to transfer her. He's just going to get advice. She shouldn't be here. She needs to be at the University of New Mexico Hospital (UNM). In a Neuroscience ICU. Where they document the Babinski. Where they can do an EEG. I thought about Regina Montoya. How they wouldn't transfer her. Even as she was deteriorating.

My first preceptor told me that the two most important things are diagnosis and treatment. You need to know what's wrong and then you need to know how to treat it. Now I believe there's another thing you need to know: who owns your hospital. It's not enough to be a good nurse, not enough to use best practice, to strive to be a good colleague to your peers, an ally to the physician, a mentor to the young, a comfort to the family. You can do all of this and fail. Because someone else may be pulling the strings.

Ardent's Code of Conduct has a section titled "Our Values." There are eight of them. Some of the values are, "We are dedicated to meeting the healthcare needs of our patients. We act with responsibility and accountability in the communities we serve. We partner with physicians to provide the best care possible for our patients." The eighth value is, "We are dedicated to providing a fair return for our investors."[3] In the world of private equity, it's called return on investment (ROI). ROI is a performance measure used to evaluate the profitability of an investment, how much investors will receive in relation to how much they invested. There's a formula. You calculate ROI by dividing net profit by the cost of investment. We don't care about that. It's not one of our values. We care about Melissa, the 42-year-old mother in room 226 whom we just diagnosed with sarcoidosis and who has an ejection fraction of 40%, who has three kids and whose husband was a long-haul trucker who died in an accident outside Tucson two years ago. We've become a different hospital since Ventas bought us. The prospectus reveals this. It is like a document you found stashed between the pages of a Mediterranean diet cookbook you never look at anymore or in a drawer with old receipts for propane and stucco work that reveals how the inheritance that was supposed to be yours was stolen or a deed that says the house you thought was yours has been sold to somebody else.

"In January 2019, the New Mexico legislature passed bipartisan Senate Bill (SB) 82, titled the Safe Harbor for Nurses Act. New Mexico Governor Michelle Lujan Grisham signed SB 82 into law on March 14, 2019."[4] According to an article by Nonnie L. Shivers and D. Trey Lynn,

> Under SB 82, a registered and licensed practical nurse may reject an assignment when he or she has a good faith belief that he or she "lacks the basic knowledge, skills or abilities necessary to deliver [safe and effective nursing care] to such an extent that accepting the assignment would expose one or more patients to an unjustifiable risk of harm or would constitute a violation of the New Mexico

Nursing Practice Act or board of nursing rules." Nurses may also reject assignments when the nurse "questions the medical reasonableness of another health care provider's order that the nurse is required to execute."[5]

Invoking safe harbor protects the patient from potential harm and protects the nurse from retaliation, demotion, suspension, termination, discipline, or being reported to the board of nursing. I think of safe harbor in an additional way. When an unqualified nurse rejects an assignment and a qualified nurse assumes the assignment, the patient is placed in a safe harbor as well. I was going to put her in safe harbor.

I go back into the room and tell the mother her daughter is having severe neurological symptoms, that she isn't getting better, that we can't provide the care she requires, and that she needs to be transferred to UNM.

"If she was my daughter, she'd be at UNM. If she was the doctor's daughter, she'd be at UNM. You need to say this to the doctor:"—I paused—"'I want to thank you for all the work you've done, and I want you to know how much I appreciate it, but I would like to have my daughter transferred to UNM.'"

She nodded.

"Can you say it?"

She looked puzzled and then smiled as if she just understood a joke. She realized I wanted her to say it, to practice.

I stood behind the hospitalist when he came into the room. He said good morning to the mother. She said good morning and then she said, "I want to thank you for all the work you've done, and I want you to know how much I appreciate it, but I would like to have my daughter transferred to UNM."

The hospitalist was quiet for a minute and then he said, in a tone that was kind and respectful, the only thing he could say: "If that's what you want, I can arrange that."

An hour later we transferred her. I helped the EMTs move her to their stretcher. They put her on their monitor. Covered her with a blanket. Strapped her in. The mother was watching. Just before they went out the door, she came up to me. She took my hand and pressed it between both of hers. She didn't say anything. I could see it in her eyes. Those tired eyes. I was glad to see the patient go because she would have a better chance at UNM, she had a mother who loved her, a child to raise, and I wouldn't come to work one day and find her dead.

Andrew Jameton writes that in situations in which nurses have ethical concerns, a secondary ethics questions arises, under the rubric of "organizational ethics": "Nurses wanting to speak with authority on ethical problems faced questions and challenges: Whom should he or she first approach—the family? The attending physician? Other nurses? A nursing supervisor? If ethical questions recur, should he or she question persistently? What is a nurse's standing as a professional to raise ethical questions in a clinical context?"[6] At Women's, you can't go to your nurse manager, the CNO, to anyone in the system. You never hear back on a MIDAS complaint. Root cause analyses don't work.

The website of the New Mexico Department of Health has a link: "Report Concerns." There's a tab to click for health facility complaints.[7] On June 29, 2019, I emailed a complaint to the Department of Health's office in Santa Fe regarding Lovelace Women's Hospital.

I wrote that I believed Lovelace Women's Hospital was a threat to public safety for the reason that the hospital was prioritizing profit over patient safety, that there was administrative interference in clinical decision-making that had led to preventable deaths over the previous 14 months. I described three incidents: the patient who was transferred from the ER to the ICU by the CNO and the house supervisor whose Levophed was not infusing, who coded on arrival in the ICU and died a week later; the

30-year-old Navajo woman who coded while restrained when the hospital failed to provide a sitter; the patient who was transferred to Med-Surg at the insistence of the CNO over the concern and objection of the charge nurse and who that evening coded and died. I requested that the New Mexico Department of Health investigate these incidents.

All Department of Health hospital surveys are unannounced. If a hospital refuses to allow immediate access for either a state agency or a Centers for Medicare and Medicaid Services surveyor, the hospital's Medicare provider agreement may be terminated. On October 29, the hospital was holding a town meeting in Auditorium B. A town meeting is where the C-team meets with the nurse managers of all the departments. It had just started when someone came in and whispered to the interim CNO that the Department of Health's survey team was in the hospital. The town meeting quickly adjourned. The survey team was in the ICU that day for four hours. They were in the hospital for three days.

On November 22, I received a letter from the manager of the Complaints Section of the Department of Health informing me that the investigation of Women's Hospital had found deficient practice and noncompliance with federal standards. A "2567" report had been issued to the facility. Centers for Medicare and Medicaid Services Form 2567 is the federal form used by the state to document inspections or surveys. It's the responsibility of the facility to respond to the 2567 form with a plan of correction. When the plan of correction is received and approved, state investigators will conduct a revisit to ensure corrections have taken place. Federal law requires that these forms be made available to the public within 90 days of a survey.

16

This Failed Practice

The 2567 report was completed on December 24, 2019. It was signed by the CEO of Lovelace Women's Hospital. The number given to the complaint was 37939. On the first page of the report, under "initial comments," is the sentence, "Complaint 37939 is substantiated with deficiencies."[1]

Each page of the 2567 report is divided into two columns side by side. The column on the left is "Statement of Deficiencies." A deficiency is a finding that a facility failed to meet a federal health requirement during an annual health inspection or a complaint inspection. The state agency completes this section.

The format is that the federal regulation the hospital failed to meet is specified—for example, "PATIENT RIGHTS: PERSONAL PRIVACY CFR [Code of Federal Regulations] 482.13 (c)(1)."[2] The report will then say, "This STANDARD is not met as evidenced by . . ." The report then details the evidence of the failure and how it was obtained, whether by review of the patient's record, by observation, or by interview.

On the right side of the page is the Plan of Correction (POC). The POC is a facility's written response to the deficiencies. The facility must respond to each deficiency and explain its plan to correct the deficiency and minimize the risk of reoccurrence.

The report is 20 pages long. The first 3 pages are definitions of terms that will appear in the report, like "intubation," "Flowsheet," "CIWA," "Code Blue," "haloperidol." Ten patients were randomly selected for review.

The first deficiency, patient #8, was "PATIENT RIGHTS: PERSONAL PRIVACY CFR: 482.13 (c) (1)."[3] The patient has the right to personal privacy. On October 29, 2019, a patient was observed in a hospital bed in front of the ER doors. He asked three different nurses to be taken to the restroom to urinate. The patient care technician gave him a handheld urinal and suggested he use it to urinate in the hallway. In an interview on October 29 at 12:00 p.m., the chief nursing officer (CNO), when asked if it was considered private to have him urinate in the hallway with only a sheet to cover him, said, "That's not private at all. That should not happen, that's not right."[4]

The second deficiency, patient #4, was "PATIENT RIGHTS: RESTRAINTS OR SECLUSION CFR 482.13 (e) (7)."[5] The attending physician must be consulted as soon as possible if the attending physician did not order the restraints. The survey found that a violent patient was placed in restraints by a nurse but there was no face-to-face assessment by the physician within one hour of the patient being placed in restraints, and the hospital failed to have the physician sign the order every four hours as required.

The remaining 14 pages are about one patient, patient #2. The patient is not identified, but by age, diagnosis, clinical course, and outcome, it is clear that it is one of the three patients in my complaint: the 30-year-old Navajo mother with a history of alcoholism who was admitted for alcohol withdrawal, was placed in restraints, suffered a cardiac arrest, was resuscitated, and, days later, was removed from life support. The report found pervasive deficiencies by the ICU nursing staff in assessing, monitoring,

documenting, administering medication, and following protocols. Failures and omissions that put the patient on a trajectory to
death.

A great deal of the deficiency section is redacted, blacked out.
Medications. Dates. "Patient was medicated with [redacted],"
"Patient was placed on [redacted]." Because what the facility
writes in the POC is cross-referenced to the deficiency, the content of the redacted material can be inferred.

The first deficiency for this patient was "PATIENT RIGHTS:
RESTRAINT OR SECLUSION CFR 482.13 (e)(16)(iv)."[6] There
must be documentation in the patient's medical record of the patient's condition or symptoms that warrant the use of restraints.

Based on record review and interview, the survey found that
there was no documentation of a comprehensive assessment or a
description of the patient's behavior that would warrant the use
of the restraints and that would have determined the most appropriate intervention necessary to effectively manage a patient
who was attempting to remove an oxygen mask and IV.

The survey team also reviewed the restraint policy at Women's
Hospital, which states that restraints are used only after alternatives have been considered or attempted. Alternatives may include
the following:

1. Reorientation
2. De-escalation
3. Increased observation or monitoring
4. Use of a sitter
5. Change in the patient's physical environment
6. Review and modification of medications regimens

The report found a failure to comply with the policy. There was
no documentation of the use of other alternatives. It also suggests
that the hospital was not forthcoming in providing the complete
patient record. The report states, "Record review of patient's

clinical record (all 659 pages provided by the facility after being asked to provide the complete record) revealed no documentation of other alternatives."[7]

The second deficiency was "PATIENT RIGHTS: RESTRAINT OR SECLUSION CFR: 482.13 (f)(2)(vi)." The hospital must require appropriate staff to have education, training, and demonstrated knowledge based on the specific needs of the patient population in at least the following: monitoring the physical and psychological well-being of the patient who is restrained or secluded, included but not limited to respiratory and circulatory status, skin integrity, and vital signs.

By record review and interview, the survey found that ICU personnel did not appropriately monitor the patient in restraints. The report discovered a course of clinical deterioration over time manifested in vital signs that were unrecognized by the ICU nurse that led to cardiac arrest. The review of the flowsheet shows vital signs—pulse, respirations, blood pressure, and oxygen level—at four times: 7:05 a.m., 11:05 a.m., 11:15 a.m., and 3:05 p.m. They are contrasted to normal ranges for the average healthy adult. The report indicates the patient was in respiratory failure. The report cites an article titled "Respiratory Failure" from MedlinePlus, which states, "Low oxygen level in the blood can cause shortness of breath and air hunger. A high carbon dioxide level can cause rapid breathing and confusion."[8]

The report then states, "On 10/30/19, the Clinical Operations Analyst confirmed that vital signs usually are taken automatically by machines in the ICU but did not necessarily mean that the nurse was at bedside and reviewing vital signs each time the machine automatically takes the blood pressure, pulse, oxygen saturation and respiratory rate."[9]

Vital signs are taken automatically by the cardiac monitor in the patient's room and sent to the electronic medical record (EMR) at variable times like 7:05 or 11:05. They appear in the EMR. By contrast, nurses who do point-of-care documentation bring their mobile computer into the patient's room, record real-time vital signs, and manually document them on the hour: 8:00, 9:00, 10:00. The times of the vital signs indicate the nurse was not at the bedside, not monitoring vital signs, not visually assessing the patient.

The patient's progressively deteriorating condition, which culminated in cardiac arrest, was not noticed by the nurse and consequently not reported to the physician. The report states there was "no documentation of care coordination with the doctor."[10] At 5:42 p.m., the nurse was called into the room by the monitor tech because the patient was in cardiac arrest. A code blue was called.

The report found a discrepancy in documentation. In the ICU, nurses document a neurological assessment every four hours. It includes level of consciousness, orientation level, and behaviors and mood. When a patient is restrained, a behavioral restraint is documented every four hours as well. It overlaps the neurological assessment and includes clinical justification, mental status, and cognitive function. The levels of consciousness in the two assessments should correspond. The survey review of the flowsheet revealed the assessments were "conflicting." Again, this suggests the nurse did not actually assess the patient.

The third deficiency was "ADMINISTRATION OF DRUGS CFR 482.23(c)(1)." Drugs and biologicals must be administered in accordance with federal and state laws, the orders of the practitioners responsible for the patient's care, accepted standards of practice, and approved medical staff policies and procedures and hospital policies.

Based on record review and interview, the survey found that the hospital failed to ensure that a patient who was receiving multiple medications that may have cumulative adverse effects was appropriately monitored and assessed according to acceptable standards of practice.

The report states the patient was started on a [redacted] protocol that requires a [redacted] medication be given as needed and that there be documentation of assessments and medication administration. In two instances, the medication was given, but there was no documentation of patient #2's [redacted] or [redacted]. Opposite this section, in the POC, is written, "As part of the Nursing Education Plan we are providing: CIWA [Clinical Institute Withdrawal Assessment for Alcohol] Protocol education for nursing in the ICU to be completed by 3/31/2020. Education on Assessment and Reassessment for pain medications to be completed by 3/31/2020."[11] The inference is that the patient was on the CIWA protocol and that on two separate occasions Ativan was given but there was no documentation of assessment or reassessment.

A record review of the patient's Medication Administration Record revealed that the patient was medicated with [redacted] at 5:32 a.m. and 9:59 the same day. At 12:07 p.m. the nurse documented that the patient was sound asleep and did not give a dose of [redacted]. The record revealed that at 2:56 p.m., 2 hours and 49 minutes after the nurse documented that the patient was sound asleep, [redacted] was administered, but there was no documentation of reassessment as to why [redacted] was given.

The report suggests the medication was the antipsychotic medication haloperidol, because immediately following the above section, the report cites an article from the *Journal of Clinical Psychology*: "Haloperidol Half-Life after Chronic Dosing": "In normal subjects, after a single dose, haloperidol half-life has been reported to range 14.5–36.7 hours (or up to 1.5 days). After chronic administration, half-lives of up to 21 days have been reported."[12]

The chronic administration of haloperidol leads to an extended half-life and a higher concentration of the drug in the body.

The report states an attempt was made to interview the nurse administering the medication, but the registered nurse was no longer employed at the facility.

On page 19, the survey reiterates that the fact that cardiac monitors in the ICU are programmed to automatically record vital signs and send them to the EMR does not mean that the nurse was at the bedside reviewing the vital signs. A record review revealed the nurses assigned to care for the patient manually time-stamped and reviewed the flowsheet records only two times, at 2:09 p.m. and at 9:25 p.m. The report concludes with a quotation from the 2019 edition of the *Lippincott Manual of Nursing Practice*: "If nonpharmacologic approaches have been applied consistently and have failed to adequately reduce the frequency and severity of behavioral symptoms that have the potential to cause harm to the patient or others, then the introduction of medications such as antipsychotics, benzodiazepines, anticonvulsants, antidepressants, and sedatives may be appropriate but will still need to be carefully and routinely monitored over time."[13]

Other factors played a part in the patient's death.

On October 31, 2019, during an interview, the quality director confirmed that the Quality Department is responsible for monitoring restraint cases and failed to do so in this case.

In the report, the CNO, on two occasions, confirms that the education and competency in restraint use had deteriorated to a substandard level.

On October 31, 2019, at 1:30 p.m., during an interview, the CNO confirmed that she was aware that the ICU staff needed additional education and training (including in the use of restraints) and an educator had been hired and had been employed in the ICU (for about a week) to ensure the nurses provided care based on standards of practice guidelines. The CNO also confirmed that the registered nurse assigned to care for the patient on the day of [redacted] was no longer employed by the facility.

On December 18, 2019, at 12:15 p.m., the CNO confirmed that staff required competency training in restraint use.

The POC is the facility's response to the deficiencies, and it lists efforts that will be taken to address them. Pages 7, 8, and 9 of the POC by Women's Hospital are blank except for the same entry on each page: "This case sent to Peer Review on 11/2/19."[14] This would be a day after the survey.

The bulk of the POC is a plan for a virtually complete reeducation and new core competency–based orientation of the emergency department and ICU nursing staff on medication administration, assessment and reassessment for pain medications, documentation of vital signs, the use of restraints, and CIWA protocol. In addition, Quality, which had been auditing pain medication since June 2019, would include assessment and reassessment as of February 2020.

On page 14 of the 2567 form, in the POC, the hospital wrote,

On or around 4/2/2019, The Quality Director called the Department of Health (DOH) to verify if we need to report this case. I was told no. The Quality Director, Risk Manager, and the House Supervisor reviewed the CMS [Centers for Medicare and Medicaid Services] requirements of reporting the death of a patient in restraints and decided the patient did not meet those requirements. The patient had been [redacted] for [redacted] hours and [redacted] minutes. According to those requirements, the patient did not meet those requirements, which are:

- Death that occurred while in restraints.
- Death that occurs within 24 hours after the patient has been removed from restraints.
- We didn't feel the [redacted] contributed directly or indirectly to the patient's death according to the CMS guidelines.[15]

The POC is referring to 42 CFR 482.13(g), "Death reporting requirements: Hospitals must report deaths associated with the use of seclusion or restraint." The regulation states,

> (1) With the exception of deaths described under paragraph (g)(2) of this section, the hospital must report the following information to CMS by telephone, facsimile, or electronically, as determined by CMS, no later than the close of business on the next business day following knowledge of the patient's death:
>
> (i) Each death that occurs while a patient is in restraint or seclusion.
>
> (ii) Each death that occurs within 24 hours after the patient has been removed from restraint or seclusion.
>
> (iii) Each death known to the hospital that occurs within 1 week after restraint or seclusion where it is reasonable to assume that use of restraint or placement in seclusion contributed directly or indirectly to a patient's death, regardless of the type(s) of restraint used on the patient during this time. "Reasonable to assume" in this context includes, but is not limited to, deaths related to restrictions of movement for prolonged periods of time, or death related to chest compression, restriction of breathing, or asphyxiation.[16]

The text in the POC is not the full section of the CFR. The hospital failed to include 42 CFR 482.13(g)(iii). The date of death is not recorded, although it is unlikely that if the family withdrew support after the cardiac arrest, it would have exceeded a week. To say of a patient who suffered a cardiac arrest while in restraints that the restraints did not contribute directly or indirectly to her death would seem untenable.

Rather than see an event such as this the way high-reliability organizations do, as a window of opportunity to improve safety and the quality of care, Ardent looks at them through an economic prism that sees investigations by government agencies as a financial threat.

The risk disclosure statement of the prospectus for the initial public offering includes the following:

> Healthcare companies are subject to various investigations and audits by governmental authorities. . . .
>
> Responding to investigations can be time and resource-consuming and can divert management's attention from the business. Additionally, as a result of these investigations, healthcare providers and entities may have to agree to additional compliance and reporting requirements as part of a consent decree or corporate integrity agreements. Any such investigation or settlement could increase our costs or otherwise have an adverse effect on our business. Even an unsuccessful challenge or investigation into our practices could cause adverse publicity, and require us to incur significant costs and could result in a material adverse effect to our reputation and business.[17]

Reported events not only invite investigations that can lead to heightened scrutiny, they can threaten reimbursement. As the prospectus observes,

> There is a trend in the healthcare industry among government, commercial and other payers towards value-based purchasing of healthcare services. Generally, value-based purchasing initiatives tie payment to the quality and efficiency of care. For example, Medicare requires hospitals to report certain quality data to receive full reimbursement updates and does not reimburse for care related to certain preventable adverse events (called "never events") or care related to hospital acquired conditions ("HACs").[18]

It also notes, "Trends toward clinical transparency and value-based purchasing may impact our competitive position and patient volumes."[19]

Hospitals that fail to report deaths related to restraints are subject to termination from the Medicare program under Section

1866 of the Social Security Act. The regulation calls for hospitals to report deaths directly to their CMS regional office, not to a state survey agency. It's not considered to be within the purview of a state agency. An Office of the Inspector General report, *Hospital Reporting of Deaths Related to Restraint*, found that state survey agencies do not provide regular guidance on the reporting requirement and fewer than 20% of state survey agencies provide information on an ongoing basis.[20]

The investigation of the death of a 30-year-old Navajo woman was like a searchlight that laid everything bare at Women's Hospital. It exposed the consequences of private equity ownership: a depleted workforce, the erosion of core competencies of nursing practice, violation of patient rights, failure to adhere to standards of care, disregard for patient safety, the vulnerability of the indigent and the innocent. When the focus of a hospital shifts away from quality of care and patient outcome to revenue generation and profit, deterioration in care, the transgression of standards, and reporting requirements are ignored.

In the Department of Health and Human Services 2567 report, a deficiency is defined as a "failed practice." The description of each one ends with a virtually identical statement on the consequences. On not documenting the patient's condition or symptom that warranted the use of restraint: "This failed practice may have contributed to further injury, additional complication, and death while a patient experiencing respiratory problems was restrained."[21] On not monitoring the physical and psychological well-being of the patient who is restrained: "This failed practice has the potential to cause further harm or complications to patients and may affect all current and future patients of the facility."[22] On failing to ensure that patients receiving multiple medications are effectively monitored and assessed: "This failed practice may cause further harm or complications to patients which may include but are not limited to drowsiness or sedation, confusion, slurred speech, respiratory depression or even death and may affect all patients in the facility."[23]

In my complaint, I wrote that I believed Lovelace Women's Hospital was a threat to public safety. I wondered then if that was an exaggeration, an overly dramatic statement. I don't think so now. The failed practice led to death.

17

Coda

Over the past two decades, private equity has begun to silently and stealthily take over health care. "PE capital invested in healthcare grew from less than $5 billion per year in 2000 to $100 billion in 2018—a 20-fold increase. Cumulatively, PE firms closed roughly 7,300 'deals' totaling $833 billion since 2000, with 70 percent of these investments occurring since 2010. In 2018 alone, PE investments in healthcare reached an historic high—at 855 deals and $100 billion in capital invested that year."[1]

Private equity companies now own rural hospitals, nursing homes, air ambulance services, fertility clinics, outpatient care centers, home health companies, addiction treatment facilities, funeral homes, ambulatory surgeries, and laboratory practices. From 2016 to 2020, private equity firms acquired 578 physician practices in dermatology, ophthalmology, and gastroenterology.[2] Private equity controls nearly half of all urgent care centers. They're involved in health-care billing and debt collection. Private equity stalks aging. In 2010, there were 28 reported private equity buyouts in elder and disabled care; in 2020, there were 61.[3] In 2021, the managing director of Provident Healthcare Partners said private equity was "bullish" on the hospice sector.[4] With $2.5 trillion in uninvested funds available as "dry powder," and the lure of federal spending on health care expected to increase 5.5% annually until 2027, private equity is poised to overwhelm health care.

Private equity may be opaque to public scrutiny and operate beneath the regulatory radar, but there is growing recognition of its harmful effects on health care in America. A May 18, 2021, report by the American Antitrust Institute (AAI), *Soaring Private Equity Investment in the Healthcare Sector: Consolidation Accelerated, Competition Undermined, and Patients at Risk,* argued that "the private equity business model is fundamentally incompatible with sound healthcare that serves patients. It is focused on short-term revenue generation and consolidation and not on the care and long-term wellbeing of patients."[5] The report argued that the proliferation of private equity investments in health care is a threat to both the structure and the goals of our health-care system. "Our healthcare system is organized on a private for-profit and non-profit basis with a professional, cultural, and legal foundation that places the well-being of patients ahead of the financial interests of the providers and organizations that compose it. There is reason for grave concern that private equity investment could tear this foundation apart."[6]

"America for Sale? An Examination of the Practices of Private Funds" was presented to the Committee on Financial Services of the US House of Representatives by Americans for Financial Reform on November 19, 2019. The testimony shined a spotlight on some of the abusive practices of private equity, which include "destroying retail jobs, saddling people with unmanageable medical bills through surprise billing, gouging students at for-profit colleges that fail to provide an adequate education, exacerbating the affordable housing crisis by buying up single-family houses, apartment buildings, and manufactured home communities after the financial crisis and raising rents and harassing tenants."[7]

Whereas private equity acquisition can lead to lost jobs, widening economic inequality, and the bankruptcy of successful businesses, in health care the consequences of the private equity business model are reduced competition and more expensive and lower-quality health care. And lost lives.

The AAI report cited a February 2021 National Bureau of Economic Research working paper, "Does Private Equity Investment in Healthcare Benefit Patients? Evidence from Nursing Homes." The study begins with the question whether the profit-driven incentive of private equity firms is misaligned with the social goal to deliver affordable, quality care. The authors study the effects of private equity ownership on patient welfare at nursing homes. Using data from the Centers for Medicare and Medicaid Services, the authors analyzed 18,485 nursing homes between 2000 and 2017. Of these, 1,674 were acquired by private equity firms in 128 deals. Over 7 million Medicare patients were observed.[8]

A key measure of patient welfare is short-term survival. The research found that private equity ownership increases the short-term mortality of Medicare patients. The likelihood of dying in a nursing home within the first 90 days of being admitted is 10% higher when the nursing home is owned by private equity. This translated into 20,150 lives lost due to private equity ownership over the sample period, more than 1,000 deaths every year. The authors estimated loss in life-years to be 160,000.[9] The study found a decrease in frontline nursing and overall staffing with consequent declines in measures of patient well-being such as decreased mobility and increased pain intensity. The study also found that going to a private equity–owned nursing home increases the probability of taking antipsychotic medications—discouraged in the elderly due to their connection with increased mortality—by 50%. The elevated use of antipsychotics often functions as a chemical straitjacket that is employed in response to lower nurse availability. Fifteen percent of the total effect on mortality is potentially attributable to starting antipsychotics.[10]

We live in era where markets and market values govern our lives. The conviction is that maximizing the reach and frequency of market transactions leads to prosperity and freedom and is the most efficient means for allocating social goods. The goal is to bring all human action into the domain of the market. If markets do not exist, they must be created. As noted by Michael J. Sandel, the author of *What Money Can't Buy: The Moral Limits of Markets*, "The reach of markets, and market-oriented thinking, into aspects of life traditionally governed by nonmarket norms is one of the most significant developments of our time."[11] Over the last two decades, private equity has methodically moved into existing market sectors such as health care, manufacturing, retail, energy, and information technology and into areas that had not been markets. The public sector, from Emergency Medical Services to municipal water systems, has become increasingly privatized. "In 1998, a national survey of cities found that not one had privatized its ambulance services. By 2012, 40% had."[12] Private equity has commodified incarceration. "Private equity-owned corporations had entered the core sectors of prison and jail operations, creating 'markets behind bars' in telecommunications, commissary sales, health provision, and a range of other services."[13]

Sandel observes that one of the tenets of market faith is that there is no moral limit to markets: "Commercializing an activity doesn't change it; money never corrupts, and market relations never crowd out non-market norms" such as altruism, generosity, benevolence, civic duty, or feelings of service or obligation.[14]

The counterargument is that markets do crowd out morals. "Market values corrupt, dissolve, or displace nonmarket norms." Markets change "the character of the goods themselves and the norms that should govern them."[15]

Laura Katz Olson writes, "Whatever PE shops take over is re-configured in their own image, engendering new language, knowledge, form, and content."[16] Private equity's transformation of health care has been moral, crowding out the benevolence, the feeling of service, the good inherent in the practice of health care.

The first modern hospice was created by Dame Cicely Saunders in 1967. From her relationship with a dying Polish refugee, she saw that terminally ill patients needed compassionate care to help allay their fears and concerns, as well as palliative treatment for physical symptoms. Her concept of "total pain" was meant to include psychological and spiritual distress as well as physical discomfort.

The hospice industry in America during the 1970s began with small nonprofit providers who relied heavily on volunteers. The mission was to care for the dying by addressing the terminally ill patient's physical pain and emotional and spiritual needs at the end of life. The 1982 Tax Equity and Fiscal Responsibility Act authorized payment for end-of-life care under Medicare and transformed hospice into a $22.4 billion industry. In 2021, almost three-quarters of the nation's 5,000-plus hospices were for-profits, many affiliated with regional or national chains. According to a 2021 analysis, "The number of hospice agencies owned by private equity firms increased from 106 in 2011 to 409 in 2019. Seventy two percent of hospices acquired by private equity were nonprofits."[17]

Private equity has reconfigured the hospice industry. Compared with nonprofit hospices, private equity–owned hospices are less likely to provide a visit to a patient in the last three days of life; less likely to provide more intense and more expensive levels of care for patients undergoing a crisis in their symptoms; tend to enroll fewer cancer patients, who have greater medical needs and usually die sooner; recruit patients with dementia, who require less care and are likely to live longer and hence are more profitable; enroll patients who are ineligible for hospice care and thus lose access to curative or emergency care; and discharge a higher number of patients before dying either because their care became more expensive or because they were enrolled without being terminally ill.

The phrase "no margin, no mission" is attributed to Irene Kraus, the nun who led the Daughters of Charity National Health System. She meant it to explain that her hospitals needed to make money and couldn't rely on charitable donations alone. Margin is the defender of the mission. Private equity has shown that, in health care, it is all margin, no mission.

If the profit-seeking goal of private equity is a threat to the mission and purpose of health care, it is also a threat to the practices of medicine and nursing, which embody and execute that mission.

As a result of private equity purchases, the percentage of doctor-owned practices has changed dramatically. The number of deals in which private equity acquired physician practices rose from 75 in 2012 to 484 in 2021. The American Medical Association reported that 2018 was the first year in which more physicians were employees (47.4%) than owners of their practices (45.9%). In 1988, 72.1% of medical practices were owned by physicians.[18] Physicians in private equity–owned firms worry about losing control of decision-making, being pressured to overprescribe diagnostic tests, or being forced to perform unnecessary procedures. The American Medical Association has warned that private equity limits the autonomy of doctors and can interfere with the doctor-patient relationship—the core of the health-care system.

Beth Israel Deaconess Medical Center in Boston is the teaching hospital of Harvard Medical School. It was formed out of the 1996 merger of Beth Israel Hospital and New England Deaconess Hospital. Dana Beth Weinberg's essay "When Little Things

Are Big Things: The Importance of Relationships for Nurses' Professional Practice," describes her fieldwork as a novice sociologist at the medical center in 1999.[19] Her interest was how the merger and subsequent budget cuts affected nurses. The research led to her book *Code Green: Money-Driven Hospitals and the Dismantling of Nursing*.[20] It documented how hospitals, driven by financial motives, were changing nurses' work and compromising their ability to provide high-quality patient care.

Beth Israel was nationally and internationally recognized as a pioneer in developing a professional model of nursing practice. It was one of the most studied nursing programs in the world. The concept was primary nursing, where the same nurse cared for the same patient from admission to discharge. It elevated the professional status of nursing by recognizing even mundane tasks as part of the complicated process of assessing patients, implementing the treatment plan, and evaluating its efficacy. Nurses, not aides, provided all aspects of care. In talking with, feeding, bathing, and toileting, the nurse gathers information and assesses the patient's response to illness and treatment. They're instrumental activities, vehicles for gathering information about the patient. Little things that enable the nurse to do big things: assess the patient, monitor progress, plan care.

An essay by Suzanne Gordon and Sioban Nelson in *The Complexities of Care* describes an ad produced by the British Columbia Nurses Union to explain the importance of nursing to the public. In the ad, a nurse is standing smiling at a patient's bedside as he is about to begin eating his hospital meal. The ad reads, "He thinks he's having a conversation about the hospital Jell-O. She's actually midway through about 100 assessments. Any one of which could mean the difference between recovery and tragedy."[21]

The new hospital, Beth Israel Deaconess Medical Center, facing a financial crisis, looked to cost-cutting. Outside consultants targeted nursing as an area for reductions. Nurses were asked to take more, sicker patients. Work with unlicensed nursing assistants. Take on tasks done by ancillary staff like blood draws, patient transport. The nurses complained to Weinberg of the diminished ability to develop relationships with patients, to gather information, to know them. With the loss of knowing, nurses become witnesses, not advocates. Private equity ends knowing.

Ardent did not disclose a reason for the withdrawal of its initial public offering, but industry recognition of its precarious financial situation fueled the decision. Moody's is an American business and financial services company headquartered in the World Trade Center. It's the holding company for Moody's Investors Service, an American credit rating agency. Credit agencies rate a debtor's ability to pay back debt and the likelihood of default. Moody's ratings system has two categories. The investment category is for financially sound companies. The speculative category is for companies with a higher risk of defaulting. Securities are assigned a rating from Aaa to C, with Aaa being the highest quality and C the lowest quality. As you move down the rating scale, default risk rises.

At the time of the initial public offering in 2018, "Moody's Investors Service assigned a Caa2 rating to $535 million of eight-year senior unsecured notes offered by Ardent. The Caa2 rating is indicative of low-quality notes that carry significant credit risk. In addition, a B3 and B1 rating, indications of speculative and high-risk characteristics, were assigned to Ardent for its $765 million senior secured term loan."[22] Moody's defines credit risk as the risk that a company may not meet its contractual financial obligations as they come due.

When Eileen Appelbaum and Rosemary Batt decided to focus their research on private equity funds in 2009, there was relatively little known about how private equity actually worked. "It was very hard for us to get access to private-equity firms," Batt wrote.

"We didn't have too many interviews. We did a lot of reading."[23] Private equity doesn't have to reveal very much. Unlike public companies, private equity companies do not have to disclose the income of their senior leaders, which companies they have in their portfolio, or financial details about them. They don't have to tell who the investors are. How much they're paying for the company. But going public changes that. A prospectus is a tell-all. Names, numbers, salaries, debts, losses, risks. The Ardent prospectus is a picture of a company that was deeply in debt, that was facing multiple threats, imminent and long term, to its solvency.

Before the purchase by Ventas in 2015, Ardent owned 14 hospitals in three states, generating $2 billion in revenue. By the end of 2020 Ardent had doubled in size, operating 31 hospitals with 26,000 employees across six states and generating $4.4 billion in revenue. AAI's 2021 report included four case studies of different segments of the health-care industry: the home health-care company Jordan Health Services, the pharmaceutical company Par Pharmaceutical, the outpatient services provided by Advanced Dermatology and Cosmetic Surgery, and Ardent Health Services as a provider of inpatient services. AAI chose Ardent as a case study because it exemplifies how private equity's debt-funded expansion strategy in the hospital industry can load the portfolio company with an amount of debt so onerous it can lead to financial crisis. AAI's report states, "Ardent's dividend recapitalizations, sale-leaseback agreement, and issuance of junk bonds are indicative of private equity firms' focus on providing investor returns. After a failed IPO, it became clear that Ardent is struggling to pay down its debts. Ardent's debt obligations may eventually overburden the system and cause the firm to start divesting facilities."[24]

I know now why worlds met. Why the world of finance in Nashville, Tennessee, appeared in the eight-bed ICU of Lovelace Women's Hospital on Montgomery Boulevard in Albuquerque,

New Mexico. How private equity changed the allegiance of executives, the way medicine was practiced, how we provided care, what we saw as our mission. Why patients died. I wrote. I laid out a line of words. It dug a path I followed. I found myself deep in new territory. I wrote about it. This writing. The hope, as the scholar David Morris wrote, is that "sometimes a single life, if sufficiently lucid, can serve as a lens to bring diffuse and complex social forces into sharper focus."[25]

NOTES

Prologue

1. Alastair V. Campbell, *Moderated Love: A Theology of Professional Care* (London: SPCK, 1984), 84.
2. Jake W. Spidle Jr., *The Lovelace Medical Center: Pioneer in American Health Care* (Albuquerque: University of New Mexico Press, 1987).
3. Annie Dillard, *The Writing Life* (New York: HarperPerennial, 1989), 3.
4. Timothy Hampton, "'Murder Most Foul' and the Haunting of America," MIT Press Reader, April 3, 2020, https://thereader.mitpress.mit.edu /murder-most-foul-and-the-haunting-of-america/.

Chapter 1. The Covenant

1. Charles Rosenberg, *The Care of Strangers: The Rise of America's Hospital System* (New York: Basic Books, 1987).
2. V. B. Price, *A City at the End of the World* (Albuquerque: University of New Mexico Press, 1992).
3. Mike Easterling, "New Mexico Again Had Third-Highest Poverty Rate in United States in 2021," *Las Cruces Sun News*, May 3, 2023, https:// www.lcsun-news.com/story/news/2023/05/03/new-mexico-continues -to-post-one-of-countrys-highest-poverty-rates/70169744007/.
4. "Albuquerque, NM," Data USA, accessed June 17, 2024, https://datausa .io/profile/geo/albuquerque-nm.
5. Susan Montoya Bryan, "Albuquerque, New Mexico, Shatters Homicide Record by 46%," AP News, January 3, 2022, https://apnews.com /article/crime-violence-albuquerque-homicide-gun-violence -247f47ccd641e8ed4cddac956e9c2dc8.
6. Rick Nathanson, "NM's Rise in Homelessness Tops Nation; HUD Reports 27% Increase in One Year," *Las Cruces Sun News*, January 14, 2020, https://www.lcsun-news.com/story/opinion/2020/01/14/27 -percent-increase-homelessness-shows-new-mexico-tops-nation /4470178002/.
7. "City of Albuquerque Acquires Gibson Medical Center, Cornerstone of Gateway Shelter Network," City of Albuquerque, April 6, 2021,

https://www.cabq.gov/mayor/news/city-of-albuquerque-acquires
-gibson-medical-center-cornerstone-of-gateway-shelter-network.
8. Price, *City*, 122.
9. *"The Myth of Santa Fe,"* University of New Mexico Press, accessed
   June 17, 2024, https://www.unmpress.com/9780826317469/the-myth
   -of-santa-fe/.
10. "Lovelace Women's Hospital," Lovelace Health System, accessed
    August 19, 2024, https://lovelace.com/location/lovelace-womens
    -hospital.

Chapter 2. Lovelace, 1922–1991
1. Erna Fergusson, *Our Southwest* (New York: Alfred Knopf, 1940), 228.
2. Jake W. Spidle Jr., *Doctors of Medicine in New Mexico: A History of Health
   and Medical Practice, 1886–1986* (Albuquerque: University of New Mexico
   Press, 1986), 94.
3. Nancy Owen Lewis, *Chasing the Cure in New Mexico: Tuberculosis and
   the Quest for Health* (Santa Fe: Museum of New Mexico Press, 2016), 127.
4. Jake W. Spidle Jr., *The Lovelace Medical Center: Pioneer in American
   Health Care* (Albuquerque: University of New Mexico Press, 1987), 14.
5. Spidle, ix.
6. Spidle, 22, 23.
7. Spidle, 22, 23.
8. Spidle, *Doctors of Medicine*, 300.
9. Spidle, *Lovelace Medical Center*, 91.
10. Spidle, 97.
11. Spidle, 100.
12. Spidle, 181.
13. Spidle, 181.
14. Spidle, *Doctors of Medicine*, 309.

Chapter 3. Private Equity
1. Eileen Appelbaum and Rosemary Batt, *Private Equity at Work: When
   Wall Street Manages Main Street* (New York: Russell Sage Foundation,
   2014), 157.
2. Steven J. Sless, "Leveraging Housing Wealth with Jumbo Reverse
   Mortgages during Economic Uncertainty," Senior Living News, April 10,
   2020, https://www.seniorlivingnews.com/leveraging-housing-wealth
   -with-jumbo-reverse-mortgages-during-economic-uncertainty/.
3. Dan Primack, "Private Equity Takeovers Result in Significant Job
   Losses," Axios, October 7, 2019, https://www.axios.com/2019/10/07
   /private-equity-employment-job-losses.

4. Doug Henwood and Liza Featherstone, "After Wall Street's Destruction of Toys 'R' Us, Pension Funds May Divest from Private Equity," *In These Times*, July 11, 2018, https://inthesetimes.com/article/toys-r-us-bankruptcy-pension-funds-divest-from-private-equity.

5. Appelbaum and Batt, *Private Equity at Work*, 15.

6. Appelbaum and Batt, 17.

7. Appelbaum and Batt, 18–19.

8. Appelbaum and Batt, 19.

9. Appelbaum and Batt, 3–4.

10. Dan Dunn, "The Private Equity Sector Sees the Return of CEO Turnover," Slayton Search, August 2021, https://www.slaytonsearch.com/2021/08/ceo-turnover-private-equity-sector-2/.

11. Appelbaum and Batt, *Private Equity at Work*, 54.

12. Appelbaum and Batt, 69.

13. Khadeeja Safdar and Miriam Gottfried, "How One Investor Made a Fortune Picking Over the Retail Apocalypse," *WSJ*, March 21, 2018, https://www.wsj.com/articles/how-one-investor-made-a-fortune-picking-over-the-retail-apocalypse-1521643491.

14. Brendan Ballou, *Plunder: Private Equity's Plan to Pillage America* (New York: PublicAffairs, 2023), 27.

15. Appelbaum and Batt, *Private Equity at Work*, 72.

16. Ballou, *Plunder*, 13.

17. "Fact Sheet: Close the Carried Interest Loophole That Is a Tax Dodge for Super-Rich Private Equity Executives," Americans for Financial Reform, October 14, 2021, https://ourfinancialsecurity.org/2021/10/close-the-carried-interest-loophole-that-is-a-tax-dodge-for-super-rich-private-equity-executives/.

18. Yves Smith, "A Bad Man's Guide to Private Equity and Pensions," Truthout, June 26, 2015, https://truthout.org/articles/a-bad-man-s-guide-to-private-equity-and-pensions/.

19. Appelbaum and Batt, *Private Equity at Work*, 83.

20. Jim Schleckser, "The 6 Things a Private Equity Firm Will Do after It Buys Your Business," *Inc.*, October 16, 2018, https://www.inc.com/jim-schleckser/the-6-things-a-private-equity-firm-will-do-after-they-buy-your-business.html.

21. Alia Paavola, "Steward Directed Staff to Delay Payments to Vendors, Former Controller Says," Becker's Hospital Review, August 6, 2020, https://www.beckershospitalreview.com/finance/steward-directed-staff-to-delay-payments-to-vendors-former-controller-says.html.

22. Heather Perlberg, "How Private Equity Is Ruining American Health Care," Bloomberg, May 20, 2020, https://www.bloomberg.com/news

/features/2020-05-20/private-equity-is-ruining-health-care-covid-is
-making-it-worse.

23. Thomas G. Wollmann, "How to Get Away with Merger: Stealth
Consolidation and Its Effects on US Healthcare" (NBER Working Paper
27274, May 2020, revised March 2024, National Bureau of Economic
Research, Cambridge, MA), https://www.nber.org/system/files/working
_papers/w27274/w27274.pdf.

24. Gretchen Morgenson and Lillian Rizzo, "Who Killed Toys 'R' Us? Hint:
It Wasn't Only Amazon," *Wall Street Journal*, August 23, 2018, https://
www.wsj.com/articles/who-killed-toys-r-us-hint-it-wasnt-only
-amazon-1535034401.

25. Rosemary Batt and Eileen Appelbaum, "Private Equity Pillage:
Grocery Stores and Workers at Risk," *American Prospect*, October 26,
2018, https://prospect.org/power/private-equity-pillage-grocery
-stores-workers-risk/.

26. Jim Baker, Maggie Corser, and Eli Vitulli, "Pirate Equity: How Wall
Street Firms Are Pillaging American Retail," July 2019, United for
Respect, https://united4respect.org/pirateequity/.

27. "Toys 'R' Us," Wikipedia, last revised August 17, 2024, https://en
.wikipedia.org/wiki/Toys_%22R%22_Us.

28. Ballou, *Plunder*, 63.

29. Tricia McKinnon, "Why Toys 'R' Us Had a Fall from Grace and Filed
for Bankruptcy," Indigo9 Digital, March 29, 2021, https://www
.indigo9digital.com/blog/privateequityinretail.

30. Sheelah Kolhatkar, "How Private-Equity Firms Squeeze Hospital
Patients for Profits," *New Yorker*, April 9, 2020, https://www.newyorker
.com/business/currency/how-private-equity-firms-squeeze-hospital
-patients-for-profits.

31. Eileen Appelbaum, "How Private Equity Makes You Sicker," *American
Prospect*, October 7, 2019, https://prospect.org/health/how-private
-equity-makes-you-sicker/.

32. Cris Barrish, "Bankruptcy Judge Approves $55 Million Sale of Hahn-
emann Residency Program," WHYY, September 5, 2019, https://whyy
.org/articles/bankruptcy-judge-approves-55-million-sale-of-hahnemann
-residency-program/.

33. "Rich Investors May Have Let a Hospital Go Bankrupt. Now, They Could
Profit from the Land," CNN, July 29, 2019, https://www.cnn.com/2019
/07/29/economy/hahnemann-hospital-closing-philadelphia/index.html.

34. Natalie Kostelni, "Hahnemann Goes Up for Sale, Billed as 'Generational Opportunity,'" NBC10 Philadelphia, July 30, 2020, https://www
.nbcphiladelphia.com/news/local/hahnemann-goes-up-for-sale-billed
-as-generational-opportunity/2485231/.

Chapter 4. Ardent, 2001–2020

1. "Sisters of Charity," New Mexico Historic Women Marker Program, accessed August 19, 2024, https://www.nmhistoricwomen.org/new -mexico-historic-women/sisters-of-charity/.
2. "Living Legacy," CommonSpirit St. Joseph's Children, accessed August 19, 2024, https://stjosephnm.org/about-us/living-legacy/.
3. "Sister Blandina's Biography," sisterblandina.org, accessed August 19, 2024, https://sisterblandina.org/sister-blandinas-biography.
4. David Weatherman, "St. Joseph Square: A Historical Landmark in Albuquerque's Health Care Past," UNM Digital Repository, May– June 1985, https://digitalrepository.unm.edu/cgi/viewcontent.cgi ?article=2288&context=nma.
5. "Modern Medicine, 1945–Now," Albuquerque Historical Society, accessed August 19, 2024, https://albuqhistsoc.org/SecondSite/pkfiles /pk133modernmedicin.htm.
6. Richard M. Scheffler, Laura M. Alexander, and James R. Godwin, *Soaring Private Equity Investment in the Healthcare Sector: Consolidation Acceler- ated, Competition Undermined, and Patients at Risk* (American Antitrust Institute, May 18, 2021), https://www.antitrustinstitute.org/wp-content /uploads/2021/05/Private-Equity-I-Healthcare-Report-FINAL-1.pdf.
7. "Nashville Company Buys Hillcrest HealthCare System," *Journal Record* (Oklahoma City, OK), May 12, 2004, https://journalrecord.com /2004/05/nashville-company-buys-hillcrest-healthcare-system/.
8. Winthrop Quigley, "A Brief History Explains the Changes at Lovelace," *Albuquerque Journal*, January 5, 2006.
9. Dennis Domrzalski, "Ardent Hospital in New Mexico Faces Probe," *Nashville Business Journal*, March 28, 2005.
10. "New Mexico's Behavioral Health Collaborative Encourages Lovelace Outpatient Behavioral Health Consumers to Transition Care," press release, New Mexico Interagency Behavioral Health Purchasing Collaborative, May 23, 2006, https://www.hsd.state.nm.us/wp -content/uploads/PressRelease/2f473c14ee654f868b5a25b3cfd15a6d /2006%20(5-23)%20LovelaceTransitionNR.pdf.
11. Quigley, "Brief History."
12. "New Mexico's Behavioral Health."
13. "New Mexico's Behavioral Health."
14. Quigley, "Brief History."
15. Quigley.
16. Jay Greene, "Leaving Lovelace?," Modern Healthcare, June 11, 2007, https://www.modernhealthcare.com/article/20070611/MAGAZINE /70608007/leaving-lovelace.
17. Greene.

18. Greene.

19. Martin Salazar, "Hospital Severs Ties with Lovelace," *Albuquerque Journal*, August 21, 2010.

20. Dennis Domrzalski, "How They Got Here: The Lovelace, ABQ Health Partners Impasse," *Albuquerque Business First*, October 26, 2012.

21. Molly Gamble, "Lovelace Health Claims New Mexico Physician Group Is Steering Patients Away," Becker's Hospital Review, October 22, 2012, https://www.beckershospitalreview.com/legal-regulatory-issues /lovelace-health-claims-new-mexico-physician-group-is-steering -patients-away.html.

22. "Lovelace Insurance Sues ABQ Health Partners," HealthLeaders Media, October 21, 2012, https://www.koat.com/article/lovelace -insurance-sues-abq-health-partners/5043668.

23. Debra Hammer, "Lovelace Health Plan Sues to Prevent ABQ Health Partners Doctors from Educating Their Patients about Network Changes," Modern Healthcare, October 22, 2012, https://www .modernhealthcare.com/assets/pdf/CH834851022.PDF.

24. Domrzalski, "How They Got Here."

25. Dennis Domrzalski, "Lovelace, Two Others Lose Appeal of State Medicaid Decision," Health Action New Mexico, May 29, 2013, https://www.healthactionnm.org/news/2013/05/24/lovelace-two -others-lose-appeal-state-medicaid-decision.

26. "Molina Healthcare to Assume Lovelace Medicaid Contract in New Mexico," Business Wire, July 3, 2013, https://www.businesswire.com /news/home/20130703005841/en/Molina-Healthcare-to-Assume -Lovelace-Medicaid-Contract-in-New-Mexico.

27. "Health Plan Ratings," NCQA, accessed August 19, 2024, https://www .ncqa.org/hedis/health-plan-ratings/.

28. "Blue Cross Blue Shield of NM Buying Lovelace Health Plan," DistilINFO, November 13, 2013, https://www.distilinfo.com/provider /2013/11/13/blue-cross-blue-shield-of-nm-buying-lovelace-health -plan/.

29. Winthrop Quigley, "Empty Beds Drive Lovelace Proposal," *Albuquerque Journal*, March 5, 2013.

30. Quigley; "Lovelace Medical Group to Drop Presbyterian Health Plan," Becker's Payer Issues, September 18, 2017, https://www.beckerspayer .com/payer/lovelace-medical-group-to-drop-presbyterian-health-plan .html.

31. "Lovelace Medical Group to Drop Presbyterian Health Plan."

32. Scheffler et al., *Soaring Private Equity*, 21.

33. Scheffler et al., 22.

34. Ardent Health Partners, Form S-1, Registration Statement, filed with the Securities and Exchange Commission on December 4, 2018, 2, https://www.sec.gov/Archives/edgar/data/1756655 /000119312518342132/d658879ds1.htm.
35. Scheffler et al., *Soaring Private Equity*, 22.
36. Bilbao Asset Management, "Ardent Health IPO Was Organized to Get Out of Debt," Seeking Alpha, December 11, 2018, https://seekingalpha .com/article/4227618-ardent-health-ipo-was-organized-to-get-out-of -debt&ved=2ahUKEwjqiKeD9eWGAxV_NzQIHbQHDGgQFnoEC BEQAw&usg=AOvVaw0R4sSprok2YChcvof5bGFw.
37. Ardent Health Partners, Form S-1, 1.
38. Ardent Health Partners, 39.
39. Julia Kagan, "What Is Asset-Based Lending? How Loans Work, Example and Types," Investopedia, updated May 15, 2020, https:// www.investopedia.com/terms/a/assetbasedlending.asp.
40. Ardent Health Partners, Form S-1, 39.
41. Ardent Health Partners, 39.
42. Ardent Health Partners, 40.
43. "Ardent to Refinance Debt via $990M Credit Facilities," *Nashville Post*, June 8, 2018.
44. Staff Reports, "Ardent to Refinance Debt via $990M Credit Facilities," *Nashville Post*, June 8, 2018, https://www.nashvillepost.com/ardent-to -refinance-debt-via-990m-credit-facilities/article_b394a570-5bb6 -5e41-ae05-fa4cbcb85e53.html.
45. "What Is Extinguishment of Bonds?," Prince Harry Memorial, January 9, 2020, https://princeharrymemorial.com/what-is -extinguishment-of-bonds/.
46. Ardent Health Partners, Form S-1, 71.
47. Bilbao Asset Management, "Ardent Health IPO."
48. Ardent Health Partners, Form S-1, 44.
49. Ardent Health Partners, 41.
50. Bilbao Asset Management, "Ardent Health IPO."
51. Bilbao Asset Management.
52. Eileen Appelbaum, "How Private Equity Makes You Sicker," *American Prospect*, October 7, 2019, https://prospect.org/health/how-private -equity-makes-you-sicker/.

Chapter 5. Moral Agency

1. Daniel F. Chambliss, *Beyond Caring: Hospitals, Nursing, and the Social Organization of Ethics* (Chicago: University of Chicago Press, 1996), 4.
2. Chambliss, 87.

3. Stuart E. Dreyfus, "The Five-Stage Model of Adult Skill Acquisition," *Bulletin of Science, Technology and Society* 24, no. 3 (2004): 177, https://doi.org/10.1177/0270467604264992.

4. Patricia Benner, *From Novice to Expert: Excellence and Power in Clinical Nursing Practice* (Upper Saddle River, NJ: Prentice Hall Health, 2001).

5. Angelo Gonzalo, "Martha Rogers: Science of Unitary Human Beings," Nurseslabs, updated on April 30, 2024, https://nurseslabs.com/martha-e-rogers-theory-unitary-human-beings/.

6. "Underlying Assumptions," *Patrica Benner's Novice to Expert* (blog), accessed August 19, 2024, http://psbennersnsgtheory.blogspot.com/p/underlying-assumptions.html.

7. Margaret Sandelowski, *Devices and Desires: Gender, Technology, and American Nursing* (Chapel Hill: University of North Carolina Press, 2000), 1.

8. Sandelowski, 180.

9. Ira Byock, *Dying Well* (Thorndike, ME: Thorndike, 1997), 62.

10. Patricia Benner, Christine A. Tanner, and Catherine A. Chesla, *Expertise in Nursing Practice: Caring, Clinical Judgment, and Ethics* (New York: Springer, 2009), 165.

11. Sanchia Aranda and Rosie Brown, "Nurses Must Be Clever to Care," in Nelson and Gordon, *Complexities of Care*, 141.

12. "Top 6 Quotes by Suzanne Gordon," A-Z Quotes, accessed June 18, 2024, https://www.azquotes.com/author/37926-Suzanne_Gordon.

Chapter 6. Do No Harm

1. Hippocrates, *Of the Epidemics* (Prato, Italy: Edizioni Aurora Boreale, 2023), 30; "Florence Nightingale Quotes," Goodreads, accessed June 18, 2024, https://www.goodreads.com/quotes/487512-the-very-first-requirement-in-a-hospital-is-that-it.

2. Ray Sipherd, "The Third-Leading Cause of Death in US Most Doctors Don't Want You to Know About," CNBC, February 22, 2018, https://www.cnbc.com/2018/02/22/medical-errors-third-leading-cause-of-death-in-america.html.

3. Charles E. Rosenberg, *The Care of Strangers: The Rise of America's Hospital System* (New York: Basic Books, 1987), 28.

4. L. T. Kohn, "Errors in Health Care: A Leading Cause of Death and Injury," in *To Err Is Human: Building a Safer Health System*, ed. Linda T. Kohn, Janet M. Corrigan, and Molla S. Donaldson (Washington, DC: National Academies Press, 2000), https://www.ncbi.nlm.nih.gov/books/NBK225187/.

5. "Ernest Amory Codman," Wikipedia, last edited March 14, 2024, https://en.wikipedia.org/wiki/Ernest_Amory_Codman.

6. "Joint Commission," Wikipedia, last edited June 11, 2024, https://en
.wikipedia.org/wiki/Joint_Commission.
7. "Joint Commission."
8. "Sentinel Event Policy and Procedures," Joint Commission, accessed
June 20, 2024, https://www.jointcommission.org/resources/sentinel
-event/sentinel-event-policy-and-procedures/.
9. Gunjan Singh et al., "Root Cause Analysis and Medical Error Prevention," National Institutes of Health, February 12, 2024, https://www
.ncbi.nlm.nih.gov/books/NBK570638/.
10. "Never Events," PSNet, Agency for Healthcare Research and Quality,
September 7, 2019, https://psnet.ahrq.gov/primer/never-events.
11. "When Hospitals and Surgery Centers Say 'I'm Sorry,'" Leapfrog
Group, accessed August 20, 2024, https://www.leapfroggroup.org
/influencing/never-events.
12. Molla Sloane Donaldson, "An Overview of *To Err Is Human*: Re-
emphasizing the Message of Patient Safety," National Institutes of
Health, 2008, https://www.ncbi.nlm.nih.gov/books/NBK2673/.
13. "Culture of Safety," PSNet, Agency for Healthcare Research and Quality,
September 7, 2019, https://psnet.ahrq.gov/primer/culture-safety.
14. Stephanie Veazie, Kim Peterson, and Donald Bourne, "Evidence Brief:
Implementation of High Reliability Organization Principles," National
Institutes of Health, May 2019, https://www.ncbi.nlm.nih.gov/books
/NBK542883/.
15. James Reason, *Managing the Risks of Organizational Accidents* (Burling-
ton, VT: Ashgate, 1997).
16. Jennifer Allyn, "Just Culture: Balancing Accountability with Quality
and Safety," Radiological Society of North America, February 18,
2019, https://www.rsna.org/news/2019/february/just-culture
-background.
17. "Just Culture," Wikipedia, last edited January 26, 2024, https://en
.wikipedia.org/wiki/Just_culture.
18. "Culture of Safety."
19. "Sentinel Event Alert 57: The Essential Role of Leadership in Developing a Safety Culture," Joint Commission, revised June 2021, https://
www.jointcommission.org/resources/sentinel-event/sentinel-event
-alert-newsletters/sentinel-event-alert-57-the-essential-role-of
-leadership-in-developing-a-safety-culture.

Chapter 7. Behind the Curtain

1. "History of the Shock Trauma Center," University of Maryland Medical
System, accessed June 20, 2024, https://www.umms.org/ummc/health
-services/shock-trauma/about/history.

2. David E. Clark, "R A Cowley, the 'Golden Hour,' the 'Momentary Pause,' and the 'Third Space,'" *American Surgeon* 83, no. 12 (December 2017): 1401–1406, https://doi.org/10.1177/000313481708301226.

3. Julie Watson, "'Climb the Airplane,' Pilot Told before California Crash," AP, October 12, 2021, https://apnews.com/article/san-diego-california-transportation-027902a900543cc45a77b121e0cbc949.

4. Nina Vadiei et al., "Impact of Norepinephrine Weight-Based Dosing Compared with Non–Weight-Based Dosing in Achieving Time to Goal Mean Arterial Pressure in Obese Patients with Septic Shock," *Annals of Pharmacotherapy* 51, no. 3 (2017): 194–202, https://doi.org/10.1177/1060028016682030.

5. Tim Porter-O'Grady and Sharon Finnigan, *Shared Governance for Nursing: A Creative Approach to Professional Accountability* (Rockville, MD: Aspen Systems, 1984).

6. Tim. Porter-O'Grady, "Shared Governance: Is It a Model for Nurses to Gain Control over Their Practice?," *Online Journal of Issues in Nursing* 9, no. 1 (January 2004): 1, https://pubmed.ncbi.nlm.nih.gov/14998345/.

7. Eileen Appelbaum and Rosemary Batt, *The New American Workplace: Transforming Work Systems in the United States* (Ithaca, NY: ILR Press, 1994), quoted in Sheelah Kolhatkar, "How Private-Equity Firms Squeeze Hospital Patients for Profits," *New Yorker*, April 9, 2020, https://www.newyorker.com/business/currency/how-private-equity-firms-squeeze-hospital-patients-for-profits.

8. Appelbaum and Batt, *The New American Workplace*, quoted in Kolhatkar, "How Private-Equity Firms Squeeze."

9. Appelbaum and Batt, *The New American Workplace*, quoted in Kolhatkar, "How Private-Equity Firms Squeeze."

Chapter 8. I'm Sorry

1. Emmanuel Levinas, *Ethics and Infinity* (Pittsburgh: Duquesne University Press, 1982), 87.

2. Joelle Baehrend, "100,000 Lives Campaign: Ten Years Later," Institute for Healthcare Improvement, June 17, 2016, https://www.ihi.org/insights/100000-lives-campaign-ten-years-later.

3. "Surviving Sepsis Campaign Guidelines 2021," Society of Critical Care Medicine, October 4, 2021, https://sccm.org/sepsisguidelines.

4. Frederick B. Rogers and Katelyn Rittenhouse, "The Golden Hour in Trauma: Dogma or Medical Folklore?," *Journal of Lancaster General Hospital* 9, no. 1 (Spring 2014): 11–13, https://www.jlgh.org/jlgh/media/journal-lgh-media-library/past%20issues/volume%209%20-%20issue%201/rogers9_1.pdf.

5. Daniel F. Chambliss, *Beyond Caring: Hospitals, Nursing, and the Social Organization of Ethics* (Chicago: University of Chicago Press, 1996), 16, 17.

Chapter 9. We Know Their Names

1. "Dissertation Success in 'Failure to Rescue,'" Penn LDI, accessed June 20, 2024, https://ldi.upenn.edu/wp-content/uploads/static-pages /50at50/dissertation-success-%E2%80%9Cfailure-rescue%E2%80%9D .html.

2. Jacy L. Henk, "Failure to Rescue: An Evidence Based Glimpse," Health eCareers, October 1, 2014, https://www.healthecareers.com/nurse -resources/nursing-news-updates/failure-to-rescue-an-evidence -based-glimpse.

3. Henk; Patricia Benner, *From Novice to Expert: Excellence and Power in Clinical Nursing Practice* (Upper Saddle River, NJ: Prentice Hall Health, 2001).

4. Patricia Benner, Christine A. Tanner, and Catherine A. Chesla, *Expertise in Nursing Practice: Caring, Clinical Judgment, and Ethics* (New York: Springer, 2009), 29.

5. Benner, Tanner, and Chesla, 43.

6. Benner, Tanner, and Chesla, 60.

7. Gooloo S. Wunderlich, Frank Sloan, and Carolyne K. Davis, eds., *Nursing Staff in Hospitals and Nursing Homes: Is It Adequate?* (Washington, DC: National Academy Press, 1996), 92, quoted in Sean P. Clarke and Nancy E. Donaldson, "Nurse Staffing and Patient Care Quality and Safety," in *Patient Safety and Quality: An Evidence-Based Handbook for Nurses*, ed. Ronda G Hughes (Rockville, MD: Agency for Healthcare Research and Quality, 2008), chap. 25, https://www.ncbi.nlm.nih.gov /books/NBK2676/.

8. Karen B. Lasater et al., "Evaluation of Hospital Nurse-to-Patient Staffing Ratios and Sepsis Bundles on Patient Outcomes," *American Journal of Infection Control* 49, no. 7 (July 2021): 868–873, https://doi .org/10.1016/j.ajic.2020.12.002.

9. Hoag Levins, "How Inadequate Hospital Staffing Continues to Burn Out Nurses and Threaten Patients," Penn LDI, January 9, 2023, https://ldi.upenn.edu/our-work/research-updates/how-inadequate -hospital-staffing-continues-to-burn-out-nurses-and-threaten-patients/.

10. Ardent Health Partners, Form S-1, Registration Statement, filed with the Securities and Exchange Commission on December 4, 2018, vii, https://www.sec.gov/Archives/edgar/data/1756655/00011931251834 2132/d658879ds1.htm.

11. Ardent Health Partners, 26–27.

12. "Don Berwick's Speech 'Many Is Not a Number,'" 123HelpMe, accessed June 20, 2024, https://www.123helpme.com/essay/Don-Berwicks-Speech -Many-Is-Not-A-D9ED9089010EF2F8.

Chapter 10. The Five Whys

1. Institute of Medicine, *Crossing the Quality Chasm: A New Health System for the 21st Century* (Washington, DC: National Academy Press, 2001), 45, quoted in Lee Ann Riesenberg, "Shift-to-Shift Handoff Research: Where Do We Go from Here?," *Journal of Graduate Medical Education* 4, no. 1 (March 2012), https://doi.org/10.4300%2FJGME-D-11-00308.1.
2. Joint Commission, "National Patient Safety Goals, 2006, Critical Access Hospital and Hospital National Patient Safety Goals," quoted in Riesenberg, "Shift-to-Shift Handoff."
3. "Sentinel Event Alert 58: Inadequate Hand-Off Communication," Joint Commission, September 12, 2017, https://www.jointcommission.org /resources/sentinel-event/sentinel-event-alert-newsletters/sentinel -event-alert-58-inadequate-hand-off-communication/.
4. Mind Tools Content Team, "5 Whys: Getting to the Root of a Problem Quickly," Mind Tools, accessed June 21, 2024, https://www.mindtools .com/a3mi0ov/5-whys.
5. "Misdirection (Magic)," Wikipedia, last edited November 14, 2023, https://en.wikipedia.org/wiki/Misdirection_(magic).
6. Eileen Appelbaum and Rosemary Batt, *Private Equity at Work: When Wall Street Manages Main Street* (New York: Russell Sage Foundation, 2014), 20.
7. Appelbaum and Batt, 20.
8. Appelbaum and Batt, 20.
9. Appelbaum and Batt, 270.
10. Ardent Health Partners, Form S-1, Registration Statement, filed with the Securities and Exchange Commission on December 4, 2018S-1, 108, https://www.sec.gov/Archives/edgar/data/1756655 /000119312518342132/d658879ds1.htm.
11. Ardent Health Partners, 109–110.
12. Appelbaum and Batt, *Private Equity at Work*, 20.
13. "Definition of Boarded Patient," American College of Emergency Physicians, last revised September 2018, https://www.acep.org/patient -care/policy-statements/definition-of-boarded-patient.
14. Jesse M. Pines, Robert J. Batt, Joshua A. Hilton, and Christian Terwiesch, "The Financial Consequences of Lost Demand and Reducing Boarding in Hospital Emergency Departments," *Annals of Emergency Medicine* 58, no. 4 (2011), https://doi.org/10.1016/j.annemergmed.2011.03.004.

15. Gretchen Morgenson and Emmanuelle Saliba, "Private Equity Firms Now Control Many Hospitals, ERs and Nursing Homes. Is It Good for Health Care?," NBC News, May 13, 2020, https://www.nbcnews.com /health/health-care/private-equity-firms-now-control-many-hospitals -ers-nursing-homes-n1203161.

Chapter 11. One Coyote

1. Paul Starr, *The Social Transformation of American Medicine: The Rise of a Sovereign Profession and the Making of a Vast Industry* (New York: Basic Books, 1982), 215.
2. Starr, 204.
3. Starr, 198.
4. Starr, 448.
5. Starr, 448.
6. Starr, 447.
7. Laura Katz Olson, *Ethically Challenged: Private Equity Storms US Health Care* (Baltimore: Johns Hopkins University Press, 2022), 10.
8. Ardent Health Partners, Form S-1, Registration Statement, filed with the Securities and Exchange Commission on December 4, 2018, vii, https://www.sec.gov/Archives/edgar/data/1756655 /000119312518342132/d658879ds1.htm.
9. James Wright et al., "Diagnosis and Management of Acute Cerebellar Infarction," *Stroke* 45, no. 4 (February 20, 2014), https://www .ahajournals.org/doi/10.1161/STROKEAHA.114.004474.
10. Hermann Neugebauer et al., "Space-Occupying Cerebellar Infarction: Complications, Treatment, and Outcome," *Neurosurgical Focus* 34, no. 5 (May 2013): E8, https://doi.org/10.3171/2013.2.focus12363.
11. Wright et al., "Diagnosis and Management."
12. Ardent Health Services, *One Person. One Moment. One Decision: Ardent Health Services Code of Conduct*, n.d., 7, https://ardenthealth.com/sites /default/files/Ardent_Code_Updates_2020-11-06.pdf.
13. Ardent Health Services, 28.

Chapter 12. The Tribe

1. "The Rise of the Patient Sitter—One of Healthcare's Most Undervalued Safety Tools," Becker's Hospital Review, February 17, 2016, https:// www.beckershospitalreview.com/quality/the-rise-of-the-patient-sitter -one-of-healthcare-s-most-undervalued-safety-tools.html.
2. Ben Unglesbee and Nicole Ault, "Is the Road to Bankruptcy Paved by Private Equity?," Retail Dive, November 9, 2018, https://www.retaildive .com/news/the-road-to-bankruptcy/540617/.

3. Ardent Health Partners, Form S-1, Registration Statement, filed with the Securities and Exchange Commission on December 4, 2018, viii, https://www.sec.gov/Archives/edgar/data/1756655/00011931251 8342132/d658879ds1.htm.

4. "Rise of the Patient Sitter."

5. Kirsten M. Fiest et al., "Long-Term Outcomes in ICU Patients with Delirium: A Population-Based Cohort Study," *American Journal of Respiratory and Critical Care Medicine* 204, no. 4 (August 15, 2021): 412–420, https://doi.org/10.1164/rccm.202002-0320oc.

6. Yanbin Pan et al., "Influence of Physical Restraint on Delirium of Adult Patients in ICU: A Nested Case–Control Study," *Journal of Clinical Nursing* 27, nos. 9–10 (May 2018): 1950–1957, https://doi.org/10.1111/jocn.14334.

7. 42 CFR § 482.13, https://www.law.cornell.edu/cfr/text/42/482.13.

8. James Reason, *Human Error* (New York: Cambridge University Press, 1990).

9. "Swiss Cheese Model," Wikipedia, last edited April 19, 2024, https://en.wikipedia.org/wiki/Swiss_cheese_model.

10. 42 CFR § 482.13.

11. 42 CFR § 482.13.

12. Luke Johnson, "Private Equity to Presidency Is a Leap," *Financial Times*, July 24, 2012, https://www.ft.com/content/467567ce-d4dd-11e1-9444-00144feabdc0.

13. Charles Rosenberg, *The Care of Strangers: The Rise of America's Hospital System* (New York: Basic Books, 1987), 39, 41.

14. "Laudato si'," Wikipedia, last edited June 7, 2024, https://en.wikipedia.org/wiki/Laudato_si%27.

15. James Salter, *Light Years* (New York: Vintage Books, 1975), 45.

16. James Agee, *Let Us Now Praise Famous Men* (Boston: Houghton Mifflin, 1988), x.

17. Agee, x.

18. Agee, xii.

19. "Leo Tolstoy Quotes," Goodreads, accessed June 21, 2024, https://www.goodreads.com/quotes/64245-a-quiet-secluded-life-in-the-country-with-the-possibility.

Chapter 13. Achilles in Vietnam

1. Christine A. Tanner et al., "The Phenomenology of Knowing the Patient," *Journal of Nursing Scholarship* 25, no. 4 (December 1993): 273–280, https://doi.org/10.1111/j.1547-5069.1993.tb00259.x.

2. Tanner et al., 274.

3. "Nursing Advocacy: The Role of Nurses Advocating for Patients," Hawaii Pacific University, August 29, 2023, https://online.hpu.edu /blog/nursing-advocacy.

4. American Nurses Association, "Code of Ethics for Nurses with Interpretive Statements," Penn Medicine Princeton Health, 2001, https://www.princetonhcs.org/-/media/princeton /documentrepository/documentrepository/nurses/code-of-ethics.pdf.

5. Tanner et al., "Knowing the Patient," 279.

6. Andrew Jameton, *Nursing Practice: The Ethical Issues* (Englewood Cliffs, NJ: Prentice-Hall, 1984).

7. Jonathan Shay, *Achilles in Vietnam: Combat Trauma and the Undoing of Character* (New York: Scribner, 1994).

8. "Moral Injury," Wikipedia, last edited June 22, 2024, https://en .wikipedia.org/wiki/Moral_injury.

9. Laura Weiss Roberts, "The Closure of Hahnemann University Hospital and the Experience of Moral Injury in Academic Medicine," *Academic Medicine* 95, no. 4 (April 2020): 485–487, https://doi.org/10.1097/acm .0000000000003151.

10. Tim Porter-O'Grady, "Shared Governance: Is It a Model for Nurses to Gain Control over Their Practice?," *Online Journal of Issues in Nursing*, 9, no. 1 (January 31, 2004), https://doi.org/10.3912/OJIN.Vol9No01 ManOS.

11. Jonathan Saltzman, "Brigham President Resigns from Moderna Board after Conflict of Interest Questions Raised," *Boston Globe*, July 30, 2020, https://www.bostonglobe.com/2020/07/30/nation/brigham -president-resigns-moderna-board-after-conflict-interest-questions -raised/.

12. Kelly Gooch, "Globe: Brigham and Women's President Sold Additional Stock before Moderna Board Resignation," Becker's Hospital Review, January 5, 2021, https://www.beckershospitalreview.com/hospital -management-administration/globe-brigham-and-women-s-president -sold-additional-stock-before-moderna-board-resignation.html.

13. Editorial Board, "Hospitals Need a Stronger Prescription for Keeping the Public's Trust," *Boston Globe*, August 24, 2020, https://www .bostonglobe.com/2020/08/24/opinion/hospitals-need-stronger -prescription-keeping-publics-trust/.

Chapter 14. Promises

1. Robert S. McPherson, "Navajo Livestock Reduction in Southeastern Utah, 1933–46: History Repeats Itself," *American Indian Quarterly* 22, no. 1/2 (Winter–Spring 1998): 1–18, https://www.jstor.org/stable/1185104.

2. Clyde Kluckhohn and Dorothea Leighton, *The Navaho* (Cambridge, MA: Harvard University Press, 1946), 100.

3. "1864: The Navajos Begin 'Long Walk' to Imprisonment," National Library of Medicine, accessed June 24, 2024, https://www.nlm.nih.gov /nativevoices/timeline/332.html.

4. Elizabeth G. Epstein and Sarah Delgado, "Understanding and Addressing Moral Distress," *Online Journal of Issues in Nursing* 15, no. 3 (September 30, 2010), https://doi.org/10.3912/OJIN.Vol15No03Man01.

5. Epstein and Delgado.

6. Simone Weil, *The Simone Weil Reader*, ed. George A. Panichas (Mt. Kisco, NY: Moyer Bell, 1977), 315.

7. "MIDAS+ System Offers Anonymous Reporting to Improve Patient Safety," Albert Einstein College of Medicine, accessed August 20, 2024, https://einsteinmed.edu/departments/medicine/news/midas -anonymous-reporting-patient-safety.html.

Chapter 15. Pentimento

1. Aimee Picchi, "Private Equity Rushed into Health Care—Now, a Nurse Warns: 'Be Scared,'" CBS News, July 29, 2019, https://www.cbsnews .com/news/private-equity-rushed-into-health-care-now-a-hospitals -fate-raises-fears/.

2. Kevin D'Mello, "Hahnemann's Closure as a Lesson in Private Equity Healthcare," *Journal of Hospital Medicine* 15, no. 5 (May 2020): 318–320, https://cdn.mdedge.com/files/s3fs-public/issues/articles/jhm01505318 .pdf.

3. Ardent Health Services, *One Person. One Moment. One Decision: Ardent Health Services Code of Conduct*, n.d., 7, https://ardenthealth.com/sites /default/files/Ardent_Code_Updates_2020-11-06.pdf.

4. Nonnie L. Shivers and D. Trey Lynn, "New Mexico's Expanded Employment Protections: The Safe Harbor for Nurses Act," Ogletree Deakins, April 9, 2019, https://ogletree.com/insights-resources/blog-posts/new -mexicos-expanded-employment-protections-the-safe-harbor-for -nurses-act/.

5. Shivers and Lynn.

6. Andrew Jameton, "What Moral Distress in Nursing History Could Suggest about the Future of Health Care," *American Medical Association Journal of Ethics* 19, no. 6 (June 2017): 617–628, https://journalofethics .ama-assn.org/article/what-moral-distress-nursing-history-could -suggest-about-future-health-care/2017-06.

7. New Mexico Department of Health, homepage, accessed June 24, 2024, https://www.nmhealth.org.

Chapter 16. This Failed Practice

1. Report in the possession of the author.
2. 42 CFR § 482.13, https://www.law.cornell.edu/cfr/text/42/482.13.
3. 42 CFR § 482.13.
4. Department of Health and Human Services, Statement of Deficiencies and Plan of Correction, Provider/Supplier/Clia Identification Number 320017, 4.
5. 42 CFR § 482.13.
6. 42 CFR § 482.13.
7. Department of Health and Human Services, Statement of Deficiencies, 10.
8. Department of Health and Human Services, 12.
9. Department of Health and Human Services, 16.
10. Department of Health and Human Services, 16.
11. Department of Health and Human Services, 18.
12. Department of Health and Human Services, 19.
13. Department of Health and Human Services, 20.
14. Department of Health and Human Services, 7, 8, 9.
15. Department of Health and Human Services, 14.
16. 42 CFR § 482.13.
17. Ardent Health Partners, Form S-1, Registration Statement, filed with the Securities and Exchange Commission on December 4, 2018, 29, 30, https://www.sec.gov/Archives/edgar/data/1756655/000119312518342132/d658879ds1.htm.
18. Ardent Health Partners, 25.
19. Ardent Health Partners, 25.
20. *Hospital Reporting of Deaths Related to Restraint and Seclusion* (Office of Inspector General, September 2006), https://oig.hhs.gov/oei/reports/oei-09-04-00350.pdf.
21. Department of Health and Human Services, Statement of Deficiencies, 7.
22. Department of Health and Human Services, 1.
23. Department of Health and Human Services, 18.

Chapter 17. Coda

1. Eileen Appelbaum and Rosemary Batt, "Private Equity Buyouts in Healthcare: Who Wins, Who Loses?," Institute for New Economic Thinking, March 25, 2020, https://www.ineteconomics.org/perspectives/blog/private-equity-buyouts-in-healthcare-who-wins-who-loses.
2. Yashaswini Singh et al., "Association of Private Equity Acquisition of Physician Practices with Changes in Health Care Spending and

Utilization," *JAMA Health Forum* 3, no. 9 (September 2022): e222886, https://doi.org/10.1001/jamahealthforum.2022.2886.

3. Richard M. Scheffler, Laura M. Alexander, and James R. Godwin, *Soaring Private Equity Investment in the Healthcare Sector: Consolidation Accelerated, Competition Undermined, and Patients at Risk* (American Antitrust Institute, May 18, 2021), 11.

4. Holly Vossel, "Private Equity Bullish on Hospice in 2021," Hospice News, February 16, 2021, https://hospicenews.com/2021/02/16/private-equity-bullish-on-hospice-in-2021/.

5. Scheffler, Alexander, and Godwin, *Soaring Private Equity Investment*, 2.

6. Scheffler, Alexander, and Godwin, 4.

7. "America for Sale? An Examination of the Practices of Private Funds," Americans for Financial Reform, November 19, 2019, 2, https://ourfinancialsecurity.org/wp-content/uploads/2019/11/AFR-Private-Funds-HFSC-Submission-11-19-2019-FNL.pdf.

8. Atul Gupta et al., "Does Private Equity Investment in Healthcare Benefit Patients? Evidence from Nursing Homes," SSRN, last revised November 16, 2020, https://papers.ssrn.com/sol3/papers.cfm?abstract_id=3537612.

9. Gupta et al., 22.

10. Gupta et al., 28.

11. Michael J. Sandel, *What Money Can't Buy: The Moral Limits of Markets* (New York: Farrar, Straus and Giroux, 2012), 7.

12. Brendan Ballou, *Plunder: Private Equity's Plan to Pillage America* (New York: PublicAffairs, 2023), 180, 181.

13. Jacob Swanson and Mary Fainsod Katzenstein, "Turning Over the Keys: Public Prisons, Private Equity, and the Normalization of Markets behind Bars," *Perspectives on Politics* 19, no. 4 (December 2021): 1247–1257, https://doi.org/10.1017/S1537592721002218.

14. Sandel, *What Money Can't Buy*, 125.

15. Sandel, 113.

16. Laura Katz Olson, *Ethically Challenged: Private Equity Storms US Health Care* (Baltimore: Johns Hopkins University Press, 2022), 10.

17. Markian Hawryluk, "Hospices Have Become Big Business for Private Equity Firms, Raising Concerns about End-of-Life Care," *Fortune*, July 27, 2022, https://fortune.com/2022/07/27/hospices-private-equity-firms-for-profit-end-of-life-care/.

18. Gretchen Morgenson and Emmanuelle Saliba, "Private Equity Firms Now Control Many Hospitals, ERs and Nursing Homes. Is It Good for Health Care?," NBC News, May 13, 2020, https://www.nbcnews.com/health/health-care/private-equity-firms-now-control-many-hospitals-ers-nursing-homes-n1203161.

19. Dana Beth Weinberg, "When Little Things Are Big Things: The Importance of Relationships for Nurses' Professional Practice," in *The Complexities of Care: Nursing Reconsidered*, ed. Sioban Nelson and Suzanne Gordon (Ithaca, NY: ILR Press, 2006), 30.

20. Dana Beth Weinberg, *Code Green: Money-Driven Hospitals and the Dismantling of Nursing* (Ithaca, NY: ILR Press, 2003).

21. Suzanne Gordon and Sioban Nelson, "Moving beyond the Virtue Script in Nursing: Creating a Knowledge-Based Identity for Nurses," in Nelson and Gordon, *Complexities of Care*, 28.

22. Scheffler, Alexander, and Godwin, *Soaring Private Equity Investment*, 22.

23. Sheelah Kolhatkar, "How Private-Equity Firms Squeeze Hospital Patients for Profits," *New Yorker*, April 9, 2020, https://www.newyorker.com/business/currency/how-private-equity-firms-squeeze-hospital-patients-for-profits.

24. Scheffler, Alexander, and Godwin, *Soaring Private Equity Investment*, 33.

25. David B. Morris, *Illness and Culture in the Postmodern Age* (Berkeley: University of California Press), 27.

INDEX

ABQ Health Partners, 51, 52–54
accreditation of hospitals, 76–77. *See also* Joint Commission
advocacy for the patient, 160–62, 212
Affordable Care Act, 89
Agee, James, 156
agency theory, 27–28
Albuquerque, 4–7; Ardent's entry into health care of, 47, 48–49; as capital of nuclear war machine, 4–5; covenant with people of, 2, 8; Dr. Lovelace's move to, 11; homeless population of, 5, 157–58; poverty and drug problems in, 5–6; spiritual and cultural heritage of, 6–7
alcoholism: among Navajo, 172; gastrointestinal bleed and, 132, 169, 184; hepatic failure and, 184, 185
alcohol withdrawal: CIWA assessment for, 133, 194, 198, 200; of Navajo woman in restraints, 147–48, 194–97; sitters unavailable for, 148–49; successful, 154–55
alignment with private equity: of acquired company's management, 128–31; of health-care leaders, 166–67
antipsychotic medication: in nursing homes, 207–8; for restrained patient, 198–99
apnea test, 142–43
apologizing to patient, 100–101
Appelbaum, Eileen, 26–28, 37, 40, 88–89, 128, 130, 212–13
Aranda, Sanchia, 73
Ardent: acquired by Ventas, 57–58, 83, 146, 189, 213; acquisitions under Ventas and EGI, 58–60; Code of Conduct on patient transfer, 146;

Code of Conduct on values and, 188–89; financial crisis of 2008 and, 56–57; financial threat of being investigated, 201–3; growth strategy of, 61; initial purchases of, 47–48; as investment, not health-care business, 149–50; Lovelace Women's Hospital owned by, 82; origin of, 46–47; renamed Ardent Health Services in 2005, 3, 48; weakened by moves between 2010 and 2017, 51–52; withdrawal of IPO, 68, 212. *See also* Lovelace Health Plan; Lovelace Health System; prospectus for Ardent's IPO
asystole, 121, 152
aviation medicine, 12–13, 15, 17–18

Babinski reflex, 187–88
Baca, Gloria, 119–23
bankruptcy in 1980s LBO movement, 23
bankruptcy of private equity investment: elimination of jobs in, 30, 32; financial crisis of 2008 and, 56; Hahnemann Hospital and, 41, 43; large grocery chains and, 37; with little at stake for general partners, 25; long-lasting effects of, 33, 36; overleveraged, 26; pension benefits and, 33; retailers and, 37–40, 149; strategic, 29; uses by private equity company, 33–34
Bataan Memorial Methodist Hospital, 14–15, 17, 20
Batt, Rosemary, 26–28, 37, 40, 88–89, 128, 130, 212–13
Begay, Amber, 147–48, 150, 152
behavioral health, 6, 46, 49–50, 149

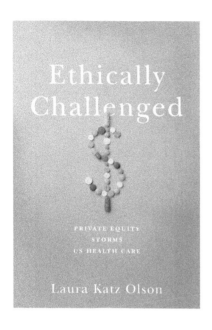
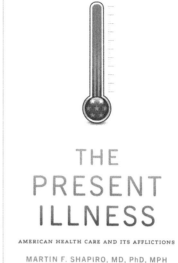

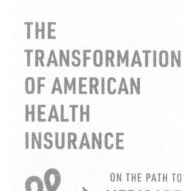
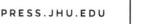